NEUROSCIENCE RESEARCH PROGRESS

SUBARACHNOID HEMORRHAGE

EPIDEMIOLOGY, MANAGEMENT AND LONG-TERM HEALTH EFFECTS

NEUROSCIENCE RESEARCH PROGRESS

Additional books in this series can be found on Nova's website under the Series tab.

Additional e-books in this series can be found on Nova's website under the e-book tab.

NEUROSCIENCE RESEARCH PROGRESS

SUBARACHNOID HEMORRHAGE

EPIDEMIOLOGY, MANAGEMENT AND LONG-TERM HEALTH EFFECTS

LINDA R. GRAY
EDITOR

NOVA BIOMEDICAL
New York

Library of Congress Cataloging-in-Publication Data

ISBN: 978-1-63463-492-2

Library of Congress Control Number: 2014955171

Published by Nova Science Publishers, Inc. † New York

Contents

Preface

Subarachnoid hemorrhage (SAH) can be classified as spontaneous or traumatic bleeding into the subarachnoid space. It is usually followed by a head injury or due to an aneurysmal rupture. Aneurysmal SAH is often a devastating occurrence that usually affects the younger population and is associated with high morbidity and mortality. Chronic smoking, heavy alcoholism, hypertension, atherosclerosis, late pregnancy are well-documented risk factors for subarachnoid hemorrhage. This book discusses the epidemiology, management and long-term health effects of subarachnoid hemorrhages.

Chapter 1 - Aneurysmal subarachnoid hemorrhage (aSAH) burdens our society not only because of its associated mortality, morbidity and disability, but also due to the high cost of treatment, rehabilitation and supportive care. After the index aneurysmal bleed, delayed vasospasm (DV) is one of aSAH's most serious complications, because it contributes to a large portion of the associated morbidity, mortality and permanent disability.

This chapter will present the evolution of the author's understanding of aSAH associated DV, including the most up-to-date concepts regarding the anatomical, physiological and molecular alterations associated with this vasculopathy, and diagnostic tools for the detection of DV. Finally, this chapter will focus on the evolution of therapeutics for the prevention and treatment of DV using an evidence-based approach.

Chapter 2 - Hydrocephalus is a common complication after spontaneous subarachnoid hemorrhage (SAH). It is seen in 15-20% of acute (48-72 hours), 2-3% of subacute (4-13 days) and 10-20% of chronic (after 14 days) cases.

SAH patients presenting with poor neurological status and presence of hydrocephalus are known indicators for adverse outcome. Although the exact mechanism for hydrocephalus remains ill-defined, leading theories include obstruction of cerebrospinal fluid (CSF) flow through the ventricles and compromised CSF reabsorption through the arachnoid granulations due to its obstruction by blood products. More recent theories propose fibrosis leading to obstruction of the fourth ventricle and arachnoid granulations, and also increased CSF production resulting in hydrocephalus. Acute hydrocephalus following SAH is usually managed by temporary CSF diversion using external ventricular drain (EVD) or lumbar drain. There are several advantages and disadvantages of the above-mentioned procedures and its placement is determined usually by patient specific issues and local practice. Above-mentioned temporary diversion procedures are gradually weaned over a period of days with the goal of discontinuation once the CSF flow dynamics have normalized. Unfortunately, guidelines are lacking regarding such weaning protocols. The number of patients who undergo permanent CSF diversion procedure is variable depending of neurosurgeons' preference that maybe based on radiological evidence of hydrocephalus versus symptomatic hydrocephalus.

Chapter 3 - The spontaneous subarachnoid hemorrhage went through different changes and developments since one of its first description by Hippocrates of Cos. The last developments in management and treatment are represented by the introduction of early intervention in aneurysms within the first 72 hours after bleeding and the introduction of endovascular coiling and stenting techniques in the 90ies. However, challenges like permanent post haemorrhage hydrocephalus, the delayed cerebral ischemia with the angiographic phenomenon of vasospasms, and cognitive deficits with impaired health-related quality of life are still present. The last and recent decade provided a sophisticated debate about the preferable treatment options within surgical and endovascular manoeuvres, especially in incidental aneurysms. When it seemed that the pendulum went to the side of endovascular treatment it recently seems to come back to surgical options. New technical achievements like neuronaviagtion and hybrid surgical theatres found the way into the field and contributed. Knowledge about the molecular and biochemical background of vasospasms and the clinical overall picture as delayed cerebral ischemia increased. This resulted in new treatment points like the continuously intra atrial given calcium channel blockers. Nevertheless, major aim is to improve the outcome for the patient with a new view including his neurocognitive and his mental conditions and to reduce his physical and psychological long term impairments.

Chapter 4 - Lumbar puncture (LP) is a safe technique used in anesthetic, diagnostic and therapeutic procedures with very few complications. Post-dural puncture headache (PDPH) is one of the commonest complications. This headache is due to leakage of cerebrospinal fluid (CSF) through dural puncture, which causes the caudal displacement of intracranial structures, leading to intracranial hypotension syndrome.

Headache is often postural with a limited time period and responds to conservative treatment. When this headache is long-lasting, it may be due to other causes like subdural hygroma, subdural hematoma, intracerebral hemorrhages (subarachnoid hemorrhage and intraparenchimal hemorrhage). Some may even appear simultaneously in the same patient or can be associated with other hemorrhagic lesions in the spinal cord (spinal epidural hematoma, spinal subdural hematoma and spinal subarachnoid hematoma (SSH)).

Subarachnoid hemorrhage (SAH) after LP is an unusual complication that requires urgent diagnosis and treatment. The physiopathologic mechanisms behind it are still not completely clear and may be multifactorial. Most presumed trigger events are associated with ruptured intracranial aneurysm, hypertensive disease, arteriovenous malformation (AVM), stress peri-anesthesia, cerebral venous thrombosis, or damaged vessels due to decreasing intracranial pressure and tractions of cerebral structures. Indeed knowing the cause of a small number of cases proves impossible.

The incidence of SAH after LP is unknown, and it is an unusual cause of PDPH after LP. Diagnosis is made according to the patient´s clinical situation, together with presence of blood in the subarachnoid space. This fact is established by a computed tomography (CT) scan that can detect most SAHs, and also helps diagnose other underlying lesions, such as intraparenchimal hemorrhage, AVM and aneurysms.

Most SAHs heal spontaneously, but can occasionally lead to death. However, it is a complication that anesthesiologists, neurologists and other specialists should take into account after LP with a severe, longer headache, or when accompanied by neurological symptoms, because early management of such complications can improve patients´ prognosis.

Chapter 5 - Subarachnoid hemorrhage (SAH) constitutes approximately 5% of all strokes and affects 21,000-33,000 people every year in the United States. Though constituting only a small proportion of incident stroke cases, SAH has a higher case fatality than other stroke types with 28-day case fatality reported as 12% for ischemic stroke, 45% for intracerebral haemorrhage, 50% for SAH and 38% for stroke of undermined type. In the absence of appropriate interventions, the number of deaths due to stroke worldwide is expected to rise to 6.5 million in 2015 and to 7.8 million in 2030. As SAH outcomes tend to change overtime, studying SAH over time is important from the stand-point of better understanding its natural course and the impact of various management strategies. Studying long-term outcomes of SAH in a population based context is important, yet there are few population based studies of SAH survivors beyond 12 months and even fewer examining wider outcomes such as neuropsychological outcomes, quality of life, disability, and mood. This chapter will review the existing literature on long-term (> 12 months) health outcomes of SAH with a focus on these less evidenced outcomes; including neuropsychological functioning, quality of life, and disability; placing these within the context of the WHO models of health.

Chapter 6 - Subarachnoid hemorrhage (SAH) can be classified as spontaneous or traumatic bleeding into the subarachnoid space. It is usually followed by a head injury or due to aneurysmal rupture. Aneurysmal SAH is often a devastating that usually affects the younger population and is associated with high morbidity and mortality. Chronic smoking, heavy alcoholism, hypertension, atherosclerosis, late pregnancy are well-documented risk factors for SAH. The basic and foremost diagnostic test includes non-contrast Computed Tomography (CT) and lumbar puncture should be performed in suspected patients with negative CT scan results. Further analysis of the underlying causes of SAH should be performed by using the digital subtraction angiography (DSA), computed tomography angiography (CTA) or magnetic resonance angiography (MRA). Patient age, level of consciousness and neurologic grading on admission are important predictive factors associated with poor prognosis after SAH. Common complications of SAH include rebleeding, vasospasm, delayed cerebral ischemia, hydrocephalus.

The most important treatment option for management of acute SAH is to stop the ongoing bleeding via immediate neurosurgical or neurointerventional procedures such as clipping and coiling. A prophylactic therapy with nimodipine has shown preventive effects so as to control the rebleeding episodes in the later phase. Early identification and prompt management of SAH is crucial for improving the prognosis.

Chapter 7 - Patients with poor-grade aneurysmal subarachnoid hemorrhage (SAH) frequently suffer devastating sequelae caused by the primary and secondary impacts on the brain, particularly if associated with large intracerebral hematoma, sylvian hematoma, or acute subdural hematoma, which result in poor outcomes due to the significant brain stem compression caused by the mass effect. The optimum treatment for aneurysmal SAH is early surgical intervention to prevent re-bleeding and for safer management of vasospasm after aneurysm obliteration. However, severe malignant vasospasm caused by SAH may develop and become resistant to conventional medical and endovascular treatments, resulting in extensive infarction and edema with secondary increased intracranial pressure (ICP) and decreased brain blood perfusion. Decompressive craniectomy (DC) is known to reduce the morbidity and mortality in critically ill patients with massive ischemic infarction and severe head injury. However, the role of DC in the treatment of SAH patients is not fully understood. Several experimental studies have indicated that DC significantly improves functional outcome due to decreased ICP or increased perfusion pressure. Clinical reports about the efficacy of DC for the treatment of poor-grade aneurysmal SAH are reviewed and discussed here.

Chapter 8 - Introduction: Volume management is crucial in intensive care, however, in some patients it is very hard to achieve optimal water balance. Subarachnoid hemorrhage (SAH) patient is a representative example. Cardiopulmonary complications are common after SAH: neurogenic pulmonary edema, cardiac failure, and so on.

Triple H therapy is a standard management after SAH, but it also has adverse effects; pulmonary edema, increased intracranial pressure, hyponatremia, sepsis and so on. The authors have just finished the multicenter prospective cohort study about cardiopulmonary function after SAH. The authors describe herein the novel goal directed therapy after SAH.

Material and Methods: This multicenter prospective cohort study analyzed the cardiopulmonary functions of 204 patients after SAH by PiCCO plus™ monitoring over a period of two weeks.

Results: Triple H therapy did not decrease the occurrence of delayed cerebral ischemia (DCI).

The risk factors of DCI on PiCCO plus™ monitoring were low cardiac index (CI), high systemic vascular resistance (SVRI), and low global end-diastolic volume index (GEDI). The cut-off value of GEDI was 822mL/m^2 to decrease the occurrence of DCI and 921 mL/m^2 to increase the occurrence of pulmonary edema.

Conclusions: Triple H therapy did not decrease the occurrence of DCI after SAH.

The authors suggested the novel goal directed therapy to prevent DCI by PiCCO plus™ monitoring. This novel goal directed therapy is to keep the GEDI between 822mL/m^2 and 921 mL/m^2.

In: Subarachnoid Hemorrhage
Editor: Linda R. Gray
ISBN: 978-1-63463-492-2

Chapter 1

Delayed Vasospasm after Subarachnoid Hemorrhage

Augusto Parra, MD, MPH, FAHA
Associate Professor, University of Texas Health Science Center - San Antonio, San Antonio, Texas, US

Abstract

Aneurysmal subarachnoid hemorrhage (aSAH) burdens our society not only because of its associated mortality, morbidity and disability, but also due to the high cost of treatment, rehabilitation and supportive care. After the index aneurysmal bleed, delayed vasospasm (DV) is one of aSAH's most serious complications, because it contributes to a large portion of the associated morbidity, mortality and permanent disability.

This chapter will present the evolution of our understanding of aSAH associated DV, including the most up-to-date concepts regarding the anatomical, physiological and molecular alterations associated with this vasculopathy, and diagnostic tools for the detection of DV. Finally, this chapter will focus on the evolution of therapeutics for the prevention and treatment of DV using an evidence-based approach.

Introduction

There are at least 20,000 aneurysmal subarachnoid hemorrhage [aSAH] cases seen per year in the U.S. Aneurysmal subarachnoid hemorrhage burdens our society not only because of its high mortality and morbidity rates, but also because of the considerable economic cost associated with treatment, rehabilitation, and supportive care. After the index aneurysmal bleed, delayed vasospasm (DV) is one of aSAH's most serious complications. It contributes to a large percentage of the adverse outcomes related to aSAH, including death and permanent disability.

The mechanisms associated with the development of DV start early, after the initial bleeding. Delayed vasospasm does not always manifest clinically, but when it does the signs and symptoms start appearing by the third day and peak by the end of the first week after the index bleeding. *The term vasospasm* implies a prolonged vascular contraction, which can lead to tissue ischemia. This definition reflects more tha acute type of vasospasm that occurs after the aneurysmal rupture. This description does not imply any vascular structural or functional changes, which are present in the delayed form.

Hippocrates could have been the first person to describe the clinical presentation of DV as a form of delayed death after a cerebral aneurysmal bleed [1]. However, Sir William Gull is the person credited for providing the first official clinic description of DV in 1859. He described a young woman suffering a stroke and her subsequent neurologic deterioration on the fifth day of her illness. Her autopsy demonstrated that she had a ruptured middle cerebral artery aneurysm [2].

Since Gull's day, there have been many advances made in the development of tools that can be used to detect DV. The ascertainment of this vascular complication was facilitated by the advent of cerebral arteriography, which was pioneered by Egas Moniz in 1927, and the development of Computerized Tomography and Magnetic Resonance angiographic techniques in the 1990's [3]. Ecker and Riemenschneider first noted the vasoconstriction of the Circle of Willis arterial branches while reviewing the angiograms of aSAH patients in 1951 [4]. Over the years we have invested a significant amount of effort into understanding the mechanisms that trigger DV, as well as the morphological and functional vascular changes associated with it. Until recently, we did not have an effective therapy to completely prevent this vascular complication of aSAH.

There are several important terms that will be mentioned in this chapter that are associated with sDV, such as delayed ischemic neurological deficit (DIND) and delayed cerebral ischemia (DCI). We will refer to DIND when discussing the clinical manifestation of sDV and DCI when referring to the radiological evidence of a stroke from sDV. Ultrasonographic thresholds (TCD mean velocities > 120 cm/sec) and angiographic reductions in diameter (< 50%) are two other concepts relevant to discussing the mechanisms of sDV.

Epidemiology

DV is a frequent and serious complication associated with aSAH. The incidence of DV associated with aSAH is about 70% (any angiographic evidence if DV), but only 20 % to 40% of those individuals suffer sDV (clinical and / or radiological manifestation of sDV) [5, 6]. In several animal models DV presentation begins during the first 24 hours, peaks at days three to four, and lasts for several days [7, 8] (Fig. 1).

In humans, DV appears on days three to four, peaks on days six to eight, and can last from 12 to 14 days after the ictus [9, 10]. There are some aSAH patients who suffer silent ischemic cerebrovascular events from DV. These events can be explained by ischemic events occurring in less eloquent areas of the brain, patient sedation, and the limited clinical assessment of severely injured patients. A clinical study by Shimoda et al., examined 165 patients with aSAH for the presence of DCI using clinical monitoring and MR brain scan assessments within three days from the onset of symptoms and at days 14 and 30 from the index event [6]. They found that DIND occurred in 38% of the group, DCI with new infarct on MRI occurred in 34%, 4% had DIND but no evidence of acute infarct on MRI, and 23% showed a new infarct on MRI (DCI) but had no clinical symptoms of sDV (DIND). Patients with DIND and new infarct on their brain MRI (DCI) had a significantly worse functional outcome than the other groups in this study. Evidence of angiographic vasospasm was seen in almost every patient with significant SAH (at least 70%).

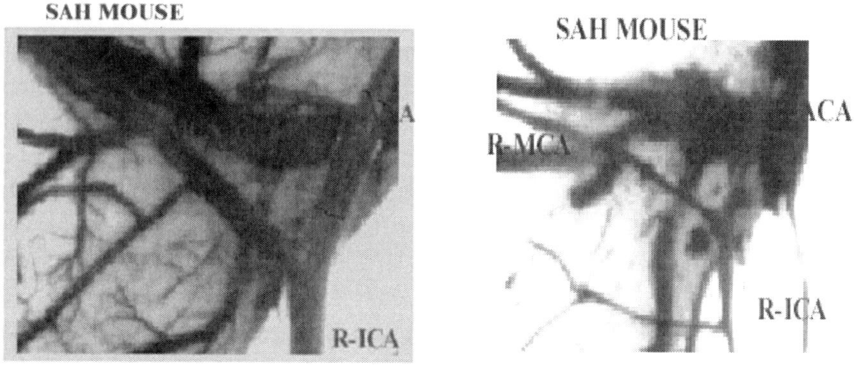

Figure 1. Mouse Endovascular Injury Model Vascular Diameter of Proximal MCA Artery: On the right normal proximal R MCA branching out of the R-ICA. On the left is the same vascular territory and using the same magnification. There is evidence of severe delayed vasospasm (3 days after SAH induction) on the R-MCA and R-ICA. (Parra et al. unpublished material).

Only 23% to 31% of aSAH cases had moderate to severe angiographic evidence of DV (< 50% narrowing of the arterial lumen) [11, 12]. The factors that influence the development of DIND and DCI are: [10]

- Extension (in the same and neighboring vascular beds) and severity of the vascular narrowing due to DV (narrowing of < 50 arterial diameter).
- Other cerebrovascular factors, such as collateral blood supply, completeness of the Circle of Willis, carotid and intracranial vascular disease, and the status of cerebrovascular auto regulation.
- Brain metabolic demand and the presence of ictal activity.
- Systemic individual factors that influence cerebral blood flow [CBF], such as systemic blood pressure, intracranial pressure, intravascular volume, cardiac output, blood viscosity and temperature.
- Medication.

The location, volume, and density of the aSAH clot can help predict the development and distribution of DV and sDV. This applies not only to humans, but also to animal models of SAH-associated DV. The proximal segments of the intracranial arteries are the segments most likely to develop DV because the bleeding aneurysm usually originates at the Circle of Willis' branching points [10].

Genetic predisposition also influences the incidence and severity of DV as well as the final outcome of aSAH patients. Genetic differences may account for a portion of the variation in the incidence of sDV among patients with similar aSAH severity [13].

The endothelial nitric oxide synthase [eNOS] gene is implicated in the development of DV. Its mutation appears to be related to the individual variability of the incidence and severity of DV. The T-786C single nucleotide polymorphism [SNP] in the eNOS gene has also been implicated in the genetic predisposition for coronary vasospasm (Prinzmetal angina) [13]. In a clinical study on aSAH patients Fisher Grade 3, this SNP of the eNOS gene was able to predict, with great accuracy, which patients would develop DV and whether or not their presentation would be severe [13]. Among the 21 patients who developed DV, 19 (90%) were cytosine allele heterozygous (T/C) and one patient was cytosine allele homozygous (C/C) for SNP of the eNOS gene. SNP with cytosine allele abnormalities was found in 57% of the patients without DV, 80% of the patients with asymptomatic cerebral vasospasm, and in 100% of the patients with sDV.

The presence of the ApoE-4 allele appears to negatively affect the overall outcome (functional and cognitive outcome) in aSAH patients [14]. Furthermore, aSAH patients with the ApoE-4 allele had more frequent sDV and were more likely to show permanent neurologic deficits in the presence of sDV than those with did not have this allele.

Haptoglobin is a two-unit peptide (alpha and beta). The gene complex for this two subunit peptide is located on chromosome 16q22. The haptoglobin alpha gene is dimorphic, encoding alpha1 and alpha-2 variants of the alpha subunit.

In a study of 32 patients with aSAH Fisher Grade 3, DV was significantly more common in patients with alpha-2 allele for the haptoglobin alpha gene than among the patients that had alpha -1 allele [13].

Delayed vasospasm can develop through other entities that cause SAH, such as traumatic brain injury, brain vascular malformation rupture, and post-surgical intracranial hemorrhage among others [10]. A study conducted on traumatic brain injury patients reported that 45.2% of the patients with TCD had mean velocities > 120 cm/s [15]. Cerebral DV after trauma has similar implications concerning the functional outcomes of patients with aSAH [15].

Angiographic arterial narrowing has been seen in other clinical entities that are not associated with SAH, such as like infectious meningitis (tuberculous and purulent meningitis), migraine, hypertensive encephalopathy, after endovascular procedures (arteriolar embolization or retrieval of an embolus), myelography, electroconvulsive therapy, and eclampsia [10].

Finally, age seems to be another factor that influences the incidence and severity of DV among aSAH patients. Younger patients appear to have a higher incidence and severity of sDV. One possible explanation for this would be that younger patients have a more robust inflammatory response to the aSAH compared to older patients [16].

Pathogenesis of Delayed Vasospasm

After the initial aneurysmal bleeding, a cascade of events begins. It includes the activation of platelets, the release of mediators (vasoactive, inflammatory and growth factor), the activation of the coagulation system, a rapid increase in intracranial pressure and the secondary cerebrovascular autoregulatory responses, direct effects of hemoglobin on the cerebral arteries, and some other direct and indirect responses to the bleeding that may ultimately end in the development of some degree of DV.

Factors that may modulate the development of DV are the individual patient's genetic characteristics, premorbid history, and the characteristics of their aneurysmal bleeding. These baseline factors also affect the patient's response to the initial aneurysmal bleeding, the development of future DV and sDV, and the long-term functional outcome.

As we described earlier in this chapter, there are two distinct types of vascular constriction that can occur after acute aneurysmal bleeding. Early vascular constriction is a hemostatic response to the bleeding. It is transient and may be driven by the release of platelet-derived vasoactive molecules, such as serotonin. This ultra-early vascular response may be involved in the early ischemic injuries seen in high-grade aSAH patients. During this chapter, we will focus on the second type of cerebral vascular constriction, delayed vasospasm (DV). Nitric oxide (NO) chelation, vascular NO depletion, free radical formation, inflammatory mediators and growth factors have all been associated with the development, severity, and duration of DV. Our current concept of DV relates more closely with delayed inflammatory arteriopathy (Fig 2).

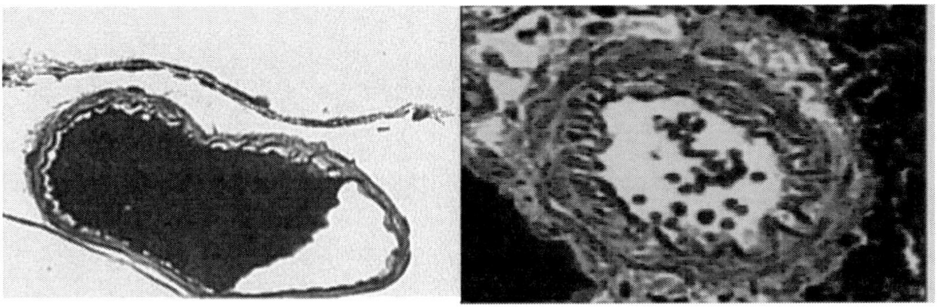

Figure 2. Mouse Endovascular Injury Model Cross Section of Proximal ACA: On the right is a normal proximal R ACA cross section. On the left is the cross section of the same vessel using the same magnification. There is evidence of severe delayed vasospasm (3 days after SAH induction) on the p-ACA. (Parra et al. unpublished material).

Hemoglobin, Nitric Oxide, and Free Radicals

SAH-associated blood products (e.g. oxyhemoglobin) are key elements in the development of delayed vasospasm. Blot clot thickness, volume, and distribution pattern are closely associated with the severity and vascular territory location of DV [9]. SAH volume, density and distance from the cerebral artery are also closely associated with the presence and severity of DV, as seen in a mouse SAH endovascular-injury model studies depicted in Table 1 and Fig. 3 [8]. That same relationship can be seen in aSAH patients.

By using SAH severity scales, we can predict the development of DV and sDV in aSAH patients. The Fisher CT Scale, the first SAH severity scale, lacked the ordinal characteristics necessary to predict the development of DV and sDV. However, the Modified Fisher Scale has an ordinal association with the development of DV. The severity of DV can be determined by giving the presence of IVH a separate score [17, 18] (Table 2). In this manner, the Modified Fisher Scale can function an independent predictor of DV [18].

Previous studies have demonstrated that erythrocytes are an integral component in the development of DV. Among them, hemoglobin appears to be the most important [19]. When compared to methemoblobin, ox-hemoglobin appears to be a more effective vasoactive agent in vitro [20].

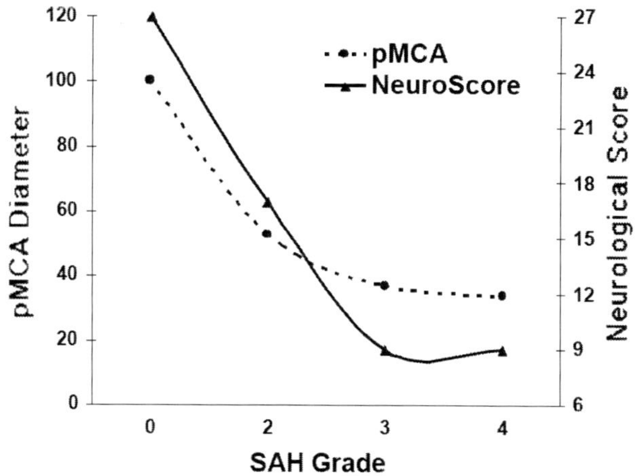

Figure 3. Mean proximal middle cerebral artery diameter (pMCA) and neurologic scores as a function of subarachnoid hemorrhage (SAH) grade. Increasing SAH grade correlated with decreasing pGMCA diameter, $p<0.01$, and decreasing neurologic score, $p<0.05$. Reproduced with permission of MANEY PUBLISHING via Copyright Clearance Center (license ID: 3512720903959)Original reference: Parra, A., et al., *Mouse model of subarachnoid hemorrhage associated cerebral vasospasm: methodological analysis.* Neurological research, 2002. 24(5): p. 510-516. (Figure 6).

Table 1. SAH Grade Score for the Mouse Endovascular Injury Model of SAH

	Extension	Density
0	No SAH	No SAH
1	< 1000 microns Anterior MCA/ACA	Transparent
2	< 1000 microns Anterior MCA/ACA	Dense
3	> 1000 microns from bifurcation but posterior and or bilateral.	

SAH grade based on density of the clot and extension from ipsilateral injury site (Parra et al., unpublished table).

NO, also known as endothelium-derived relaxing factor (EDRF), is derived from arginine by eNOS isoforms in the vascular endothelium. NO induces vascular smooth muscle relaxation by upregulating intracellular levels of cyclic guanine monophosphate (cGMP) through the activation of guanylate cyclase [21]. High intracellular cGMP in the vascular smooth muscle cell (vSMC) inhibits intracellular calcium influx, hyperpolarizes the cell by activation of the potassium channels, and induces dephosphorylation of myosin by myosin light chain phosphatase, which is activated by a cGMP-dependent kinase. All these reactions are mediated by endothelial NO and result in vasodilation. Other processes in which NO plays a modulating role are platelet activation and cell proliferation. A decrement in the production of endothelial NO or an increase in the consumption of this molecule will promote the development of DV.

Table 2. Comparison in the Frequency of DIND Between the Fisher CT Score and the Modified Fisher CT Score

Fisher CT Score	Criteria	Modified Fisher CT Score	Criteria	Fisher's DIND (%)	Modified Fisher's DIND (%)
N/A		0	No SAH or IVH	N/A	0
1	None	1	Minimal / thin SAH without IVH in the lateral ventricles	5	12
2	Diffuse layer only	2	Minimal / thin SAH with IVH in the lateral ventricles	14	21
3	Thick clot or layer	3	Thick SAH without IVH in the lateral ventricles	27	19
4	Diffuse or non with ICH and /or IVH	4	Thick SAH with IVH in the lateral ventricles	25	40

The Modified Fisher CT Scale shows a more ordinal relationship with DIND compared as compared with the Original Fisher CT Scale.

Modified Table from Claassen et al 2001.

Claassen, J., G. L. Bernardini, et al. (2001). Effect of Cisternal and Ventricular Blood on Risk of Delayed Cerebral Ischemia After Subarachnoid Hemorrhage: The Fisher Scale Revisited. Stroke 32(9): 2012-2020.

Oxyhemoglobin contributes to the development of DV by lipid peroxidation through free radical formation, direct chelation of vascular NO, and prostaglandin synthesis [22]. The breakdown of oxyhemoglobin to methemoglobin is thought to release superoxide anions (a powerful free radical), which rapidly reacts with NO to form peroxynitrite, a more potent free radical [22]. The detection of nitrothyrosine in the MCA vascular adventitia and endothelial layer of ipsilateral middle cerebral artery of a mouse SAH endovascular-injury model suggests that NO degradation to peroxynitrite and subsequent vascular oxidative injury occur after the experimental induction of SAH [22]. This free radical production consumes NO and induces cellular membrane lipid peroxidation, which causes cellular dysfunction. Endothelial dysfunction secondary to free radical related injury can decrease the production of vascular NO, which is also known as the NO sink phenomenon.

The reaction of NO with extracellular oxyhemoglobin probably accounts for most of the NO depletion [23]. The depletion of NO shifts the balance of vascular tone toward vasoconstriction [22]. Extracellular superoxide dismutase (EC-SOD) is a very potent, endogenous free radical scavenger that is located in the arterial intimal extracellular matrix [22]. EC-SOD can aid in sparing endothelial NO by shifting the superoxide reaction to form hydrogen peroxide (H_2O_2) instead of peroxynitrite. DV attenuation with an excess production of EC-SOD has been demonstrated by using transgenic EC-SOD overexpressors in mice and inducing cerebral SAH with the endovascular injury method [22].

Genetic Modifiers

ApoE is a polymorphic protein that has three common isoforms (apoE2, apoE3, and apoE4). It is a product of alleles ε2, ε3, and ε 4 at a single gene locus on chromosome 19 [14]. That peptide is produced in the central nervous system and is involved in neurotrophic (neuroplasticity and membrane repair) and neuroprotective (antioxidant activity) functions. ApoE is also involved in the modulation of the immune response. Although the *ApoE4* allele appears to be less effective than the other two alleles in fulfilling these functions, it is also associated with the modulation of endothelin-1-mediated vasoconstriction [14].

The gene encoding eNOS (7q35-36) is polymorphic in humans and the presence of T-786C single nucleotide polymorphism (SNP) in the eNOS gene increases the risk for DV in humans [13]. This SNP is associated with a significant reduction in eNOS gene promoter activity [13].

Haptoglobin polymorphism is also implicated in the development of DV. Haptoglobin containing the alpha-2 subunit is less capable of inhibiting hemoglobin-induced, free radical production, so it induces inflammation in in-vitro studies. In clinical studies, patients with the alpha-2 allele had a higher incidence of DV than those individuals with the alpha-1 allele [24].

Vascular Changes, and Growth Factors

Delayed vasospasm induces structural and functional changes in affected cerebral arteries. Macroscopically, the arteries lose their normal red appearance and have a whiter color instead. Microscopically, the affected arteries have *sustained smooth muscle contraction*. Intraluminally, there are platelet aggregates, microthrombi, or distal embolization [25]. There is evidence of delayed proliferation of myo-intimal cells and extracellular matrix in the tunica intima. The vascular segments affected by DV show smooth muscle and myofibroblast proliferation, cellular necrosis and remodeling, intimal hyperplasia, collagen deposition, and fibrosis. All these structural changes may contribute to arterial wall thickening, decreased vascular compliance, and a decrease in vascular diameter. The critical vascular diameter threshold that causes flow failure and induces ischemia is < 50% of the original diameter [10]. At that point the patient show clinical symptoms, also called DIND. This observation also holds in SAH animal models. (Fig. 4) In a mouse SAH endovascular-injury model, narrowing the proximal MCA vascular diameter < 50% was associated with motor dysfunction [22]. Delayed vasospasm, of either regional or global involvement, promotes the dysfunction of normal cerebrovascular autoregulation and subsequently reduces CBF in the more affected vascular beds [10].

The coagulation of blood in the subarachnoid space activates platelets which, in turn, release potent vasoactive molecules, inflammatory mediators and growth factors [26]. Platelet-derived growth factor-AB (PDGF-AB), transforming growth factor-β1 (TGF- β1), and vascular endothelial growth factor (VEGF) are all released by the activated platelets. The PDGFs and TGF-β1 are potent mitogens for smooth muscle cells in the vascular media and fibroblasts in the adventitia, whereas VEGF stimulates the proliferation of vascular endothelium. Previous studies have shown an increase in platelet-derived growth factor cerebrospinal fluid (CSF) titers among patients with aSAH [26]. PDGF-AB concentrations in CSF from SAH patients were significantly greater than in non-SAH patients and control group patients at each time period that was measured, including the first week after SAH.

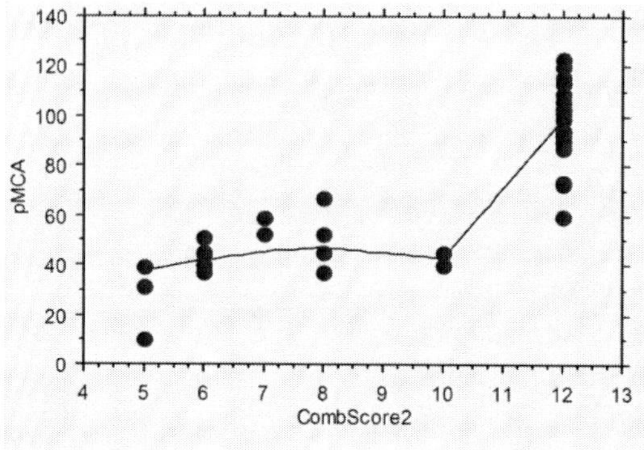

Figure 4. Mouse SAH Endovascular –Injury Model: Proximal MCA Diameter and Neurologic Motor Scores Composite Motor and Sensory Score (medianIQR) Versus Proximal MCA (pMCA) Diameter Three Days after SAH. Lower scores represent decreased motor/sensory deficits. A score of five represents a complete loss of motor and sensory function contralateral to the vasospastic MCA. Analysis of all animals revealed that neurological deficits worsen as pMCA diameter decreases. pMCA vascular diameter ranged between 110 to 90 microns. Neurological deficits worsened primarily between 70 and 50 microns (SAH mice with sDV). (Parra el a unpublished graph).

PDGF-AB and VEGF concentrations in CSF increased during the first two weeks and gradually decayed after the third week after aSAH onset (Table 3). Using immunohistochemistry techniques in conjunction with a mouse endovascular injury model, researchers were able to show evidence of cellular proliferation among the SAH-induced subjects using PCNA, a nuclear cyclin involved in DNA replication. There was an increased number of PCNA-positive perivascular nuclei among SAH animal subjects compared to the sham-injury subjects and control group. The majority of PCNA-positive nuclei were from fibroblasts located in the adventitia and connective tissue surrounding the vessels as well as a few from smooth muscle cells [26]. Smooth muscle PCNA-positive cells were in significantly higher numbers among SAH-induced subjects than in sham-injury or control subjects [26].

A thrombus in proximity to human cerebral vessels in vitro can also stimulate vascular cell proliferation (Fig. 5). The researchers were able to block this vascular proliferation by introducing inhibiting concentrations of antibodies with PDGF [26]. Their study demonstrated vascular proliferation in both mouse and human arteries.

Table 3. Growth Factor Concentrations in CSF

Patient Group	N	Peak PDGF-AB pg/ml	Peak VEGF pg/ml	bFGF pg/ml
SAH Patients				
• All Time points	14	293 +/- 232*	90 +/- 127	3.9 +/- 10.2
• First 7 days	11	322 +/- 252*	101 +/- 135	N/A
Non-SAH Patients	6	81 +/- 94	19 +/- 22	3.5 +/- 3.8
Normal Controls	8	18 +/- 6	13 +/- 9	0 +/- 0.1

Values are means SD. *P0.003 for comparisons of SAH patients, non-SAH patients, and controls. Modified table from Borel et al 2003. Borel, C.O., et al., Possible Role for Vascular Cell Proliferation in Cerebral Vasospasm After Subarachnoid Hemorrhage. Stroke, 2003. 34(2): p. 427-433.

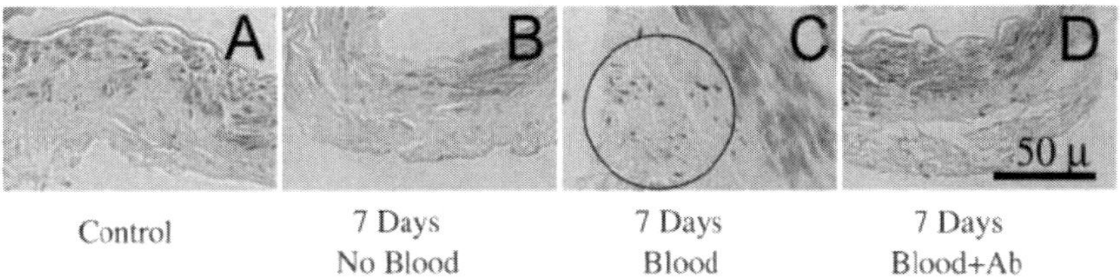

Figure 5. Human pial arteries. Representative samples of pial arteries stained for PCNA. A, Freshly excised vessel, not cultured. B, Vessel cultured for 7 days with no thrombus. C, Vessel cultured for 7 days in contact with human blood. Area of adventitial proliferation is indicated by circle. D, Vessel cultured in contact with human blood mixed with anti-PDGF antibodies. Nonspecific cytoplasmic staining of muscular layers is apparent in A, C, and D. Reproduced with permission of Walter Kluwer Health via Copyright Clearance Center's Rights Link (license ID: 3520861309575). Original reference: Borel, C.O., et al., Possible Role for Vascular Cell Proliferation in Cerebral Vasospasm After Subarachnoid Hemorrhage. Stroke, 2003. 34(2): p. 427-433. (Figure 4).

Microthombosis and Coagulation

After acute SAH, there is an activation of the coagulation cascade and an impairment of the fibrinolytic cascade. The levels of platelet-activating factor (PAF) increase within four days after the ictus which, in turn, increases platelet activation and adhesion. Elevated titers of von Willebrand factor, D-dimers, fibrin degradation products, and tissue factor in CSF are predictors of the future development of sDV, cerebral infarction, and a poor functional outcome [9]. Clinical studies using trans-cranial Doppler (TCD) in aSAH patients have detected micro-emboli in a high percentage (70%) of patients with a non-significant trend toward an increased incidence of micro-emboli in those patients who went on to develop sDV [27]; [9].

Endothelins and Prostaglandins

Hemoglobin-induced free radical injury and NO depletion appear to alter the normal balance between vasodilator and vasoconstrictor molecules such as prostacyclin, nitric oxide, endothelins, and eicosanoids in the arterial wall. The activation of inflammatory cascades with secondary vascular injury may further contribute to the imbalance of vasodilator and vasoconstrictor mediators [10].

Endothelin -1, a potent, endogenous vasoconstrictor, is up-regulated after aSAH and peaks three to four days after bleeding. Endothelin-1 mediates calcium-dependent and independent vasoconstriction via protein kinase C (PKC). Endothelin-1 is produced by the vascular endothelium and plays a role in the regulation of arterial vascular tone. It is thought to be up-regulated by the inflammatory cascade, ischemia, and other stress mediators produced after aSAH. It decreases endothelial NO levels through a negative feedback loop in eNOS activation. Endothelin-1 also plays a role in inflammation, tissue proliferation, and fibrosis. All these mechanisms, including those that generate SAH-induced NO, are mediated by endothelin-1 and may lead to sDV. Immunomodulation agents, such as trehalose, modulate the effects of the cyclooxygenase-2 (COX-2) catalytic pathway and endothelin-1. They have been shown to reverse experimental DV in SAH models [28]. The CONSCIOUS clinical trials assessing the effect of Clazosentan, an endothelin-1 inhibitor, showed that the drug significantly improved angiographic DV, but had minimal effect on neurological function [29]; [21].

Other Inflammatory Mediators

After the aneurysmal rupture, a cascade of reactions activates that includes the release of pro-inflammatory mediators and up-regulation cell adhesion molecules.

An early increase in tumor necrosis factor-α (TNF-α), interleukin-6 (IL-6), and interleukin-receptor antagonist have all been documented in both the serum and CSF of patients after SAH. These increases correlate with acute sDV, and poor functional outcomes [9, 30]. The elevation of these cytokines and the up-regulation of cell adhesion molecules (CAMSs) produces the activation, margination, rolling, endothelial adhesion, and transmigration of leukocytes into the vascular wall. This process allows leukocytes to bind to the endothelial cells and enter the subarachnoid space, where they phagocytize extravasated RBCs and process released hemoglobin. After two to four days, these cells begin to degranulate. They release large quantities of endothelins and oxygen free radicals, which results in further inflammation and possible arterial vasoconstriction. Myeloperoxidase (MPO) is a leukocyte lysosomal enzyme that catalyzes the production of hypohalous acids like hypoclorous acid, which can modify tissue membranes. Lim et al., reported elevations of MPO in CSF that mirror the onset of CBF abnormalities associated with DV after induced SAH [29, 31].

An increase in interleukin-1β [IL-1 β], IL-6, TL-8, TNF-α, and C-reactive protein (CRP) levels has been associated with experimental SAH and post-induced injury outcomes.

Bowman et al., demonstrated a significant dose-dependent reduction in DV after administration of a polyclonal antibody targeted against IL-6 [32].

In a canine SAH model, the peak expression of interleukin-1 (IL-1), IL-6, IL-8, and ICAM-1 was seven days after SAH, which correlated with the maximal arterial narrowing of angiography [33]. TNF-α is released by circulating macrophages after they are exposed to hemoglobin and activate toll-like receptor 4. Induced, direct vasoconstriction via Rac-1 activation is very likely to be involved in the development of DV [34].

Cortical Spreading Depression

Cortical spreading depression (CSD) comprises a depolarization wave in the cerebral cortex that propagates across the brain at rate of 2–5 mm/min and results in the depression of evoked and spontaneous EEG activity [35]. This phenomenon has been implicated in several neurological disorders, including malignant stroke, migraine headaches, traumatic brain injury, and sDV after SAH. Over the last few years the there has been a degree of interest in determining whether or not CSD is involved in the development of sDV [9].

Other Hemodynamic Factors

Neurogenic stunning of the myocardium (NSM) can present in patients who suffered an aSAH. It is usually seen in high-grade, young, female patients. Patients who have an acute and serious left ventricular (LV) dysfunction have been implicated in early deaths after aSAH. The effects of NSM have been studied in a well-characterized subgroup of aSAH patients [36].

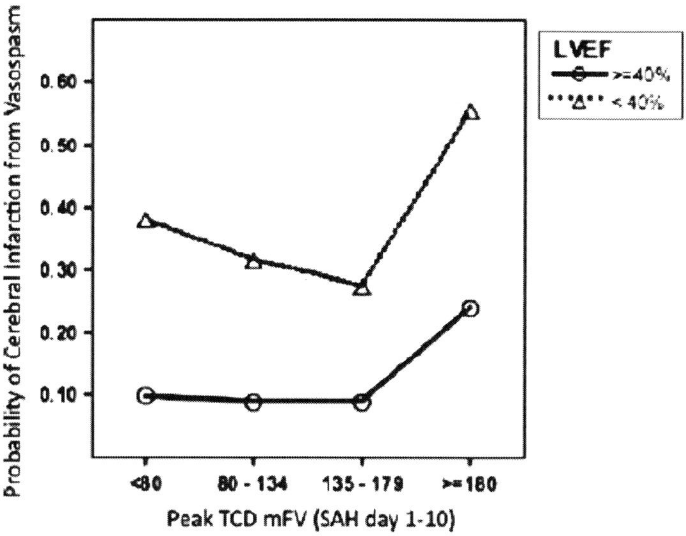

Figure 6. Risk of cerebral infarction from vasospasm as a function of peak TCD mFV during the first 10 days after SAH, divided into quartiles. For each TCD quartile, the risk of infarction is higher when LVEF is <40%; the highest risk is among those with a peak TCD mFV >180 cm/s. Reproduced with permission of Springer Science+Business Media Tiergartenstr. 17 , 69121 Heidelberg, Germany. Original reference: Temes, R.E., et al., *Left ventricular dysfunction and cerebral infarction from vasospasm after subarachnoid hemorrhage.* Neurocritical care, 2010. 13(3): p. 359-365. (Figure 1).

LV dysfunction (LV ejection fraction < = 40%) occurred in 11% of patients. A similar frequency of NSM has been reported in other groups of SAH patients, ranging from 3% to 22%. Younger age, untreated hypertension, thick clots in the 4th ventricle and quadrigeminal cistern, and acute hydrocephalus were associated with LV dysfunction. LV dysfunction after aSAH has been shown to significantly increase the probability of cerebral infarction from vasospasm [36] (Fig. 6).

Clinical Presentation, Monitoring, Diagnosis and Impact

Clinical Presentation

There are two distinct types of vascular constriction that appear after the aneurysmal rupture. Each displays a different pathophysiology. Early ischemic brain injury after aSAH has been demonstrated in up to 86% of Hunt-Hess Grades 4 and 5 patients in studies using diffusion-weighted imaging (DWI) MRI techniques [37]. (Fig. 7) Similar studies reported 79 % of patients with DWI lesions, and 76% of patients with lesions on fluid-attenuated inversion recovery FLAIR [38].

The most common patterns of injury seen were both DWI- and FLAIR-positive lesions. The average ischemic lesion was 4cc in volume. High-grade aSAH patients (Hunt-Hess 4-5) had 18-fold larger ischemic lesion volumes when compared to lower grade hemorrhages (Hunt-Hess 1-3) [38]. These early ischemic injuries could derive from hypoperfusion secondary to early intracranial hypertension (following a massive ICP surge and intracranial circulatory arrest) and/or from ultra–early vasospasm. Some experimental animal models show a biphasic pattern of vasospasm. Ultra-early vasospasm that occurs at ictus of aSAH can be regional or generalized, but is usually transient. One study using a rat SAH model showed that ischemic lesion volume on an ADC map increased between 1 and 48 h, which was attributed to early vasospasm and later confirmed on 3-dimensional MR-angiography [39]. In an SAH -dog model, this ultra –early arterial vasoconstrictive response started minutes after the induction of the SAH and remained active for less than one hour [7]. Vasoactive substances released from platelets immediately following aneurysmal bleeding, such as serotonin, may participate in this hemostatic response.

Delayed vasospasm, on the other hand, is a more complex vascular dysfunction. With DIND, vSMC starts presenting after days three to four, peaks from days eight to ten, and subsides before day 14 post-aSAH. It is rare to find sDV after day 14 post–sSAH (sDV occurs < 4% after day 13 post–aSAH) [40]. (Fig. 8 and 9) Patients who develop sDV are usually younger, have a higher grade SAH (Fisher and Modified Fisher Scales), have a larger bleeding aneurysm (higher Fisher and Modified Fisher Grades), and have a poorer neurological function on admission (lower Glasgow Coma Scores [GCS]). Symptoms of DIND can start suddenly or manifest insidiously.

A drop in blood pressure sometimes triggers the onset of symptoms. Fever and hyponatremia can precede the onset of sDV symptoms (DIND). Depending on the affected cerebral vascular beds, the patients can present with lethargy and progressive confusion with or without focal neurologic deficits. A high proportion of patients have radiological vasospasm (70%), but the majority of them are asymptomatic [40].

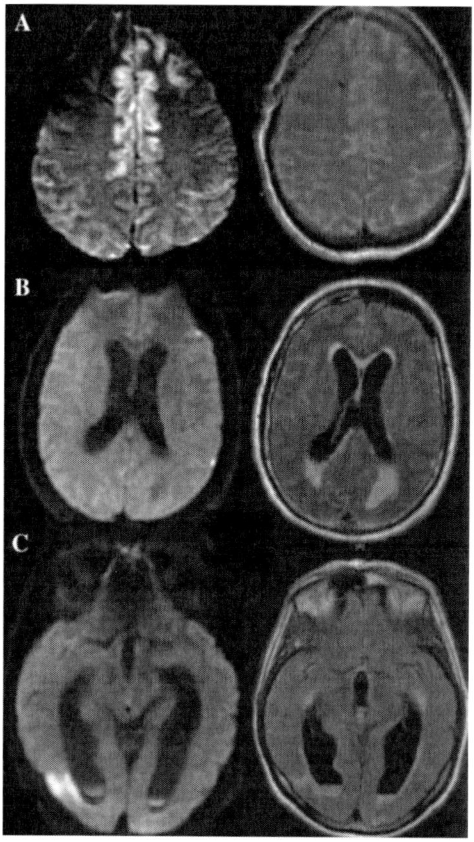

Figure 7. Common patterns of brain injury. A Displays bilateral injury to anterior cerebral artery territories visible on both diffusion-weighted imaging (DWI) and fluid-attenuated inversion recovery (FLAIR); B Displays hydrocephalus and periventricular injury on FLAIR but not on DWI, and displays a punctate DWI lesion in the left parietal cortex; C Displays patchy injury to the right temporo-occipital junction on both DWI and FLAIR. Reproduction permission from Springer. Original reference: De Marchis, G., et al., *Brain Injury Visible on Early MRI After Subarachnoid Hemorrhage Might Predict Neurological Impairment and Functional Outcome.* Neurocritical Care, 2014: p. 1-8. (Figure 1).

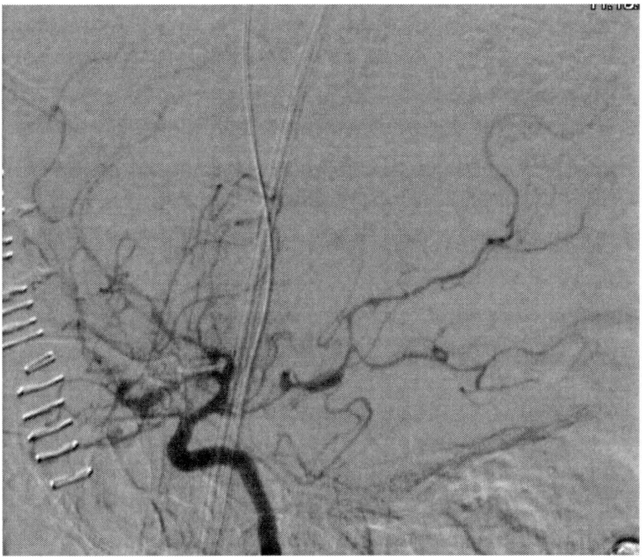

Figure 8. Severe anterior Circulation Delayed Vasospasm: 44 year old male who suffered an acute aSAH from a 7 mm Acom Aneurysm. He developed sDV and on agiography diffuse and severe vasospasm on all on his right MCA and ACA. (Parra et al. unpublished material).

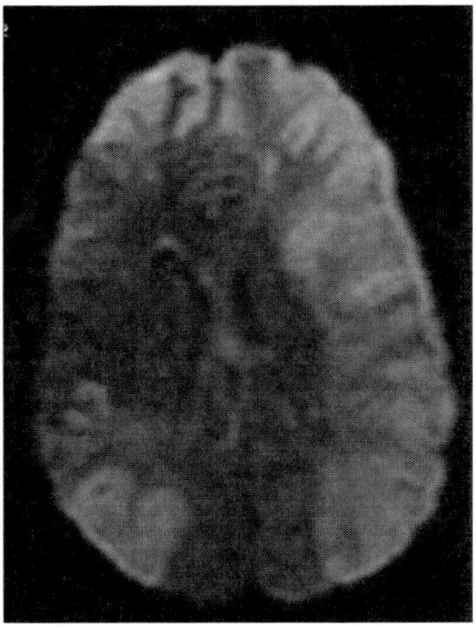

Figure 9. Left and Right MCA and ACA territory cortical strokes from Severe Delayed Vasospasm. 44 year old male who suffered an acute aSAH from a 7 mm Acom Aneurysm. He developed sDV and on agiography diffuse and severe vasospasm on all on his right MCA and ACA. (Parra et al. unpublished material).

A smaller proportion of patients (20%-40%) demonstrate symptomatic delayed vasospasm (sDV), which is the development of acute neurological deficits due to cerebral ischemia that is usually associated with a severe narrowing of the arterial lumen (<50%) [40].

The definition of sDV varies among different studies. Some definitions are clinically-based. Others are more rigorous and add a confirmatory test (e.g., cerebral angiography, a threshold on TCD mean velocities, CT angiography (CTA), and MRI/MR angiography [MRA]). Some of the considerations for the definition of sDV are: [12]; [9]

- Focal neurological signs and/or the deterioration of consciousness
- Exclusion of any other possible cause of the neurological function deterioration (e.g., aneurysmal clipping or coiling, hydrocephalus, metabolic derangements, seizures, infection, brain sagging form, lumbar drain related drainage, and oversedation)
- Duration of the neurological symptoms. Many definitions range between one to six hours. Some definitions have a duration that is less than one hour, but because clinicians intervene in these cases by augmenting the cerebral perfusion and reverting the clinical symptoms, it would not be advisable to use that range as a specific time threshold.
- New infarction on CT or MR of the brain, excluding other possible etiologies (e.g. coiling or clipping of the aneurysm, embolism from vascular dissection caused during angiography).
- Angiographic vasospasm defined as moderate to severe and arterial narrowing not present in the initial angiographic study, excluding other causes (e.g. atherosclerosis, catheter-induced spasm, vascular hypoplasia). A decrease in arterial diameter >50% is usually associated with DIND. Extension (in the same and neighboring vascular beds) and severity of the vascular narrowing from DV are also factors to consider.
- TCD mean flow velocities. TCD vasospasm was defined as a mean flow velocity in any vessel > 120 cm/sec. This cut-off point is used frequently in the literature.

The following is a proposed definition for DV that summarizes some of the previously mentioned concepts [9, 12].

Neurological Deterioration Associated with sDV (DIND)

- Focal neurological signs (such as hemiparesis, aphasia, apraxia, or neglect) and/or the deterioration of the level of consciousness (a decrease of at least 2 points on the Glasgow coma scale, either on the total score or on one of the components).
- Exclusion of any other possible cause of the neurological function deterioration (e.g., aneurysmal clipping or coiling, hydrocephalus, metabolic derangements, seizures, infection, brain sagging form, lumbar-drain related drainage, oversedation, etc.) (Table 4).
- B- New Ischemic Lesion on CT/MRA associated with sDV (DCI).
- New infarction on CT or MR of the brain, excluding other possible etiologies (e.g. coiling or clipping of the aneurysm, embolism from vascular dissection caused during angiography).
- The evidence must not be present on the CT or MRI scan between 24 and 48 hours after early aneurysm obliteration therapy (coiling or clipping) and must not be attributable to other causes (e.g. hypodensities on CT imaging resulting from ventricular catheter or intraparenchymal haematoma).

Diagnosis and Monitoring

Aneurysmal SAH patients are usually monitored for up to two weeks in a Neuro-ICU by staff members who are specially trained in clinical neuro-assessment, as well as the monitoring and treatment of SAH.

During clinical assessment, patient sedation is minimized to the lowest possible level needed for comfort; sometimes it is held off entirely. Periodic TCD assessments aid in the detection of patients who are at higher risk of developing sDV and help to identify when the DV is resolving. TCD assessments can also be used to monitor the development of arterial vasospasm (Class IIa; Level of Evidence B) [41].

When new symptoms suggestive of sDV occur, a clinician must rapidly discard other potential differential diagnosis and immediately order the needed confirmatory tests. If sDV is a likely scenario, a trial of stepwise hemodynamic augmentation should not be delayed.

Table 4. Differential diagnosis of delayed neurological deterioration after SAH

Type:	Specific Causes of Delayed Neurological Deterioration:
Neurologic	• Aneurysmal rebleeding • Epidural hemorrhage • Subdural hemorrhage • Intraventricular hemorrhage • Hydrocephalus. • Postoperative hemorrhage • Meningitis / ventriculitis • Seizures / Post-ictal starte
Iatrogenic	• Medication related 4
Electrolytes	• Hypo or hypernatremia.
Arterial Blood Gases	• Hypoxia. • Hypercapnia.
Infection	• Pneumonia • UTI • Ventriculitis / meningitis • Other infections
Other	• Fever
Cardiovascular	• Hypotension • Hypovolemia • Heart failure • Arrythmia

Modified table from MacDonald's & Peerles. (Adapted from Peerless, 1979
Modified table from MacDonald et al 2006. MacDonald, R.L., Management of cerebral vasospasm. Neurosurgical review, 2006. 29(3): p. 179-193.

Confirmatory diagnostic tests for dVS are TCD, CT angiography (CTA), and/or CT perfusion (CTP). Perfusion imaging with CT or magnetic resonance can be useful to identify regions of potential brain ischemia (Class IIa; Level of Evidence B) [41]. Cerebral angiography is usually done when the process is refractory to medical therapy and there is a need for endovascular therapy for refractory sDV (e.g. intra-arterial calcium channel blocker infusion, percutaneous angioplasty etc.). In general, the sensitivity of TCD for diagnosis of sDV is 50% to 60% for mean velocities greater than 120 cm/s to 150 cm/sec with a specificity over 90% [42]. In vascular imaging, a reduction of < 50% the cerebral artery diameter is highly associated with sDV.

Impact of Symptomatic Delayed Vasospasm

In general, more than 70% of patients develop some degree of DV after acute aSAH, 20% to 40% develop sDV, and 50% of those who develop sDV die or are left with permanent disability associated with cerebral ischemia [12]; [10]. In a cooperative study on the timing of aneurysm surgery (N= 3,521 patients), 26% of patients died or were disabled. In this portion of the population, 28% of the deaths and 39% of the disabilities were attributed to sDV [10]. In her study of sDV using clinical brain imaging, arteriographic, and TCD criteria, Frontera et al., found that 16% of her cohort of 580 aSAH patients had clinical symptoms associated with sDV (DIND), 21% had a new stroke on CT/MRI attributable to sDV (DCI), 31% had moderate to severe angiographic vasospasm, and 45% had TCD mean velocities > 120 cm/sec, which are highly associated with sDV [12]. From all the patients who had been clinical diagnosed with sDV, 85% had angiographic and 81% had TCD criteria for sDV. In her study, only DIND and DCI were significantly associated with worse instrumental activities of daily living (Lawton instrumental activities of daily living scale), cognitive impairment (telephone interview of cognitive status), and worse quality of life (sickness impact profile) after adjusting for baseline predictors of outcome (Table 5). Silent infarctions found on CT/MRI also contributed independently to a poor outcome.

Table 5. Effect of Symptomatic Vasospasm, Delayed Cerebral Ischemia, Angiographic Vasospasm, and TCD-Defined Vasospasm on Outcome

	Symptomatic Delayed Vasospasm			Delayed Cerebral Ischemia (DCI)			Angiographic Vasospasm			TCD Vasospasm		
Outcome	N(%)	aOR) (95% CI)	*P*	N(%)	aOR) (95% CI)	*P*	N(%)	aOR (95% CI	*P*	N(%)	aOR (95% CI	*P*
mRS 6	19(20)	1.1 (0.6 - 2.2)	0.751	31(26)	1.6 (0.9 - 3.0)	0.124	25 (14)	0.9 (0.4 - 2.0)	0.892	36 (14)	1.3 (0.7 - 2.4)	0.451
mRS 4-5	27 (28)	1.3 (0.7 - 2.5)	0.360	44(36)	2.2 (1.2 - 3.9)	0.007	36 (20)	1.0 (0.5 - 2.1)	0.910	53 (20)	1.4 (0.8 - 2.5)	0.232
Lawton IADL Scale >=9	48 (51)	1.9 (1.1 - 3.6)	0.031	56(46)	1.8 (0.1 - 3.2)	0.032	70 (39)	1.2 (0.7 - 2.2)	0.451	102 (39)	1.0 (0.7 - 1.7)	0.849
TICS <= 30	23 (24)	2.5 (1.1 - 5.6)	0.027	26(22)	2.7 (1.3 - 5.9)	0.011	35 (19)	1.8 (0.8 – 3.9)	0.155	47 (18)	1.2 (0.6 - 2.2)	0.653
SIP Total >=15.5	42 (44)	1.9 (1.0 - 3.6)	0.048	51(42)	2.3 (1.3 - 4.2)	0.006	67 (37)	0.9 (0.9 - 2.9)	0.136	95 (36)	1.1 (0.7 – 1.8)	0.639

IADL indicates independent activities of daily living; mRS, modified Rankin scale; SIP, sickness impact profile; TICS, telephone interview of cognitive status. mRS adjusted for age, Hunt-Hess, and aneurysm size. SIP adjusted for Hunt-Hess, race, and education. TICS adjusted for Hunt-Hess, race, age, and education. Lawton adjusted for Hunt-Hess, race, and education. Modified table from Frontera et al 2009. Frontera, J.A., et al., *Defining Vasospasm After Subarachnoid Hemorrhage What Is the Most Clinically Relevant Definition?* Stroke, 2009. 40(6): p. 1963-1968.

The incomplete correlation between clinical and angiographic moderate to severe vasoconstriction-associated DIND could be related to impairment at the microvascular level. Hypovolvemia and hyponatremia are particularly problematic in this patient population. Hyponatremia, if caused by cerebral salt wasting, is accompanied by hypovolemia.

Therapeutic Approaches

General Recommendations

Patients who are at a higher risk of developing sDV should be monitored for at least 10-14 days in a specialized Neuro-ICU. It is recommended that this patient population avoid hypotension, hyperthermia, hyperglycemia, hypovolemia, hyponatremia, hypomagnesemia, increased intracranial pressure, seizures, hypercapnia, and hypoxia. Non-invasive hemodynamic monitoring is also recommended for aSAH patients. Central venous access should be started in unstable and high-risk patients as per clinical criteria. The patients should have euvolemic maintenance and fluid restriction ought to be avoided during the sDV monitoring period. External ventricular drainage is recommended if there is evidence of hydrocephalus. Clamping trials should be avoided during the peak days for the onset of sDV, especially if TCD mean velocities are elevated. Sedation should be minimized and, if feasible, periodic clinical assessment should be performed during sedation-free intervals. Increased intracranial pressure should be treated as per standard of care; prolonged elevations of ICP above 20 mmHg, especially if CPP are < 60 mmHg, should be avoided. Prolonged hyperventilation with significant hypocapnia (PaCOs< 30 mmHg) should be avoided since it can induce cerebral ischemia. Antiepileptics are not recommended after aneurysmal clipping unless the patient has evidence of seizures or significant cortical irritability. Steroids are not recommended in general for these patients unless they suffer severe pain from chemical meningitis.

Clot removal, Intra-thecal Thrombolysis, and Lumbar Cerebrospinal Fluid Drainage

Animal and clinical studies suggest that removing the clot can help in the prevention of DV [43, 44]. The impact of clot removal is greater if it is done early after the hemorrhage. The effects are similar to those if intracisternal fibrinolysis with tissue plasminogen activator in animal models [45]. Surgical clot removal is technically difficult and often done in an incomplete fashion. In a clinical trial of perioperative, post-aneurysmal obliteration, some researchers had the idea of infusing intracisternal or intraventricular fibrinolytic to dissolve and drain the SAH clot. A double-blind, placebo-controlled trial was done to test the impact of intrathecal thrombolysis on the functional outcome. The favorable outcomes were slightly higher among the treated subjects, but they were statistically non-significant [46]. On the other hand, Hamada et al., did a clinical study using intrathecal urokinase in the cisterna magna after aneurysm coiling [47]. No serious complications were reported. Symptomatic delayed vasospasm (sDV) was reduced from 30% to 9% in the patients who received urokinase. This study has not yet been replicated elsewhere.

Subarachnoid blood drainage using a lumbar drain has also been studied as a method to ameliorate or prevent DV. The LUMAS trial evaluated 210 patients with aSAH. 105 were randomized to receive standard therapy and a lumbar drain while the other 105 were randomized to the control group and received only standard management [48]. As of day 10 post-SAH, the authors found a significant reduction of sDV and improved, early functional outcomes using the modified Rankin Score (mRS). These results were not still visible at 6 months. The EARLYDRAIN study still needs to evaluate this type of therapy as a reliable means of preventing sDV [49].

Hemodynamic Augmentation

Formerly, the artificial elevation of blood pressure, the increase in intravascular volume, and the reduction of blood viscosity and optimization of cardiac output in order to increase CBF was called triple–H therapy. This therapy was initially used in a preventative manner, but after a randomized and blinded clinical study that compared normovolemia to hypervolemia for 14 days after aSAH, the use of hemodynamic augmentation as a prophylactic, especially with hypervolemia, was discontinued. There was no effect on CBC and no decrease in the incidence of sDV among the treated patients [50]. Euvolemia is recommended during the whole observation period and hemodynamic augmentation with stepwise blood pressure elevation is advisable only when sDV is present. The induction of hypertension is recommended for patients with DCI unless their blood is elevated to baseline pressure or their cardiac status precludes it. Class I; Level of Evidence B) [41].

Hypervolemia appears to show an increase in cardiopulmonary complications like pulmonary edema. Hypertensive hemodynamic augmentation is safe to use in order to treat sDV only when the bleeding aneurysm is adequately obliterated. Hemodilution is not recommended because there is no evidence of its efficacy. The hemoglobin level should be kept around 10 mg/dl (Hct over 30%). There is ongoing research assessing the ideal hemoglobin threshold for this patient population.

Pharmacologic Therapy

Calcium Channel Blockers

Nimodipine prophylaxis is the only pharmacologic therapy that is highly recommended by the American Heart Association Guidelines and Neurocritical Care Society Guidelines for the management of aSAH. Oral nimodipine should be administered to all patients with aSAH (Class I; Level of Evidence A). [41, 51]. Nimodipine is a voltage-gated calcium channel antagonist that inhibits calcium entry into vascular smooth muscle and neurons. There is significant evidence of its efficacy from eight randomized placebo-controlled trials. A meta-analysis of seven nimodipine trials found that nimodipine improved the odds of a good outcome by 1.86 and reduced the odds of deficit and/or mortality due to sDV and infarction on CT scan (DCI) by 0.46 to 0.58 [52]. Nimodipine had no statistically significant impact on mortality. Not all the clinical trials demonstrated that the drug successfully ameliorated DV in arteriography. The main limitation with this treatment is hypotension. Nimodipine may exert its major protective effect through calcium inhibition in neurons [10]. On the other hand, nicardipine, another dihydropyridine, appears to show a more robust effect in treating angiographic DV. This could be explained, in part, because some of the studies testing the drug used it at higher doses than the ones that studied nimodipine. Selective intra-arterial infusions of nicardipine are currently being used for the treatment of refractory DIND; they show promising efficacy.

Amino Steroids

Tirilazad (U74006F) is a 21-amino steroid that was developed with the intention of inducing anti-inflammatory and anti-oxidant effects without the glucocorticoid side effects of steroids. It has been the subject of four randomized, placebo-controlled double-blind studies (N=3,500 patients). This medication is approved for use in some countries but not in the United States of America. A meta-analysis of these studies suggested that the drug was effective in a subgroup of patients composed of poor-grade SAH males [53].

Fasudil

Fasudil (AT877 or HA1077) is a protein kinase inhibitor that inhibits multiple kinases including rho kinase, which decreases smooth muscle contractibility [54]. Rho kinase increases the smooth muscle contractile apparatus to calcium. The main clinical trial studying this molecule was carried out in Japan using patients with aSAH (N=276 patients) [55]. Fasudil significantly reduced DIND from 50% (placebo group) to 35% (treatment group), but had no significant effect on outcome. It is currently used in Japan to treat aSAH patients.

Endothelin Antagonists

There is preclinical evidence that endothelins appear to be involved in the development DV. TAK-044, an antagonist of A and B endothelin receptors, was clinically tested in a placebo-controlled trial (N=420 patients). The therapy (or placebo) was started within 96 hours from the onset of the aSAH. {Shaw, 2000 #237}. It did not prevent DIND, nor did it have any significant effect on patient outcome. The patients in the treatment arm had significantly more hypotension compared to the control group. Another placebo-controlled trial using a selective endothelin A receptor called Clazosentan was also completed (N=32) [56]. Clazosentan was shown to be effective in preventing angiographic DV (88% in placebo vs. 40% in the treated patients). Furthermore, the severity of vasospasm was reduced after selective intra-arterial infusions of Clazosentan by cerebral angiography. This study was followed by the CONSCIOUS 1,2, and 3 randomized placebo-controlled trials for Clazosentan. CONSCIOUS-2 tested Clazosentan infusion at 5mg/hr, against a placebo. The CONSCIOUS-3 trial tested three arms of treatment consisting of 5mg/hr, 15mg/hr, and a placebo for 14 days post-aSAH [57]. CONSCIOUS-3 was halted prematurely following the completion of CONSCIOUS-2. Only 38% of the planned study population was enrolled and 571 were treated (placebo, N=189; Clazosentan 5 mg/h, N= 194; Clazosentan= 15 mg/h, B=188). The primary composite end point (all-cause mortality, vasospasm-related new cerebral infarcts or delayed ischemic neurological deficits, and rescue therapy for vasospasm) was evaluated six weeks post-aSAH. The main secondary end point was dichotomized using the extended Glasgow Outcome Scale at 12 weeks. Clazosentan was effective in reducing the composite primary outcome at the dose of 15mg/hr (OR, 0.474; 95% CI,

0.275– 0.818; P= 0.007). Unfortunately, the Clozasentan group had increased pulmonary complications, anemia, and hypotension compared to the placebo group. That group also had a non-significant trend for worse functional outcome at 12 weeks using the Glasgow Outcome Scale. The medication had no significant effect on mortality. The study was stopped abruptly for safety reasons; nevertheless, the drug appeared to have some significant effects on the sDV-related outcome components.

Magnesium

Magnesium is a non-competitive, voltage-dependent calcium channel antagonist with vasodilator and neuroprotective effects in animal models [58]. It induces vasodilatation by blocking the voltage-dependent calcium channel, decreases glutamate release, and reduces calcium entry into cells [59]. Furthermore, magnesium may attenuate the vasoconstrictor effect of endothelin 1 and block the formation of oxygen-derived free radicals. There is preclinical support for the use of magnesium as a neuroprotective and/or vasodilatory agent in SAH patients.

There have been six phase II trials. Most were small and had a negative primary outcome. One of the larger trials showed a significant reduction in sDV by one third, but had a negative primary endpoint (hypodense lesion on CT) [60]. MASH –II is currently in the works. It is a phase III randomized, clinical international multicenter trial comparing magnesium sulfate (16 gr/day) vs placebo within 4 days of the hemorrhage until day 20 post-SAH. The primary outcome measure is poor (Rankin score >3), which is defined as death or dependence after 3 months. Its planned study population is 1200. Given the inconsistency of the clinical trial results, the recommendation regarding magnesium is to correct aggressive hypomagnesaemia when present, but to avoid the regular use of high magnesium concentration drips for neuroprotection and/or the prevention or treatment of sDV [51].

Statins

Statins have pleiotropic biological properties with modulatory effects on the immune response and up-regulation of eNOS, which are key mechanisms in the development of DV. Statins appear to have a positive effect on the amelioration of DV in the mouse endovascular injury model. The effect is more robust if it is given before or shortly after the induced hemorrhage (Fig. 10 and 11) [61]. There appears to be a short window of time during which it can affect some of the cascades derived from the induced SAH. The first clinical study regarding patients already on statins at the time of the hemorrhage used a matched retrospective cohort design [62]. The patients already on statins had significantly less DV and sDV (DIND) as well as fewer strokes associated with sDV (DCI). (Fig. 12) Statin-user patients had significantly lower peak TCD mean velocities compared to the controls.

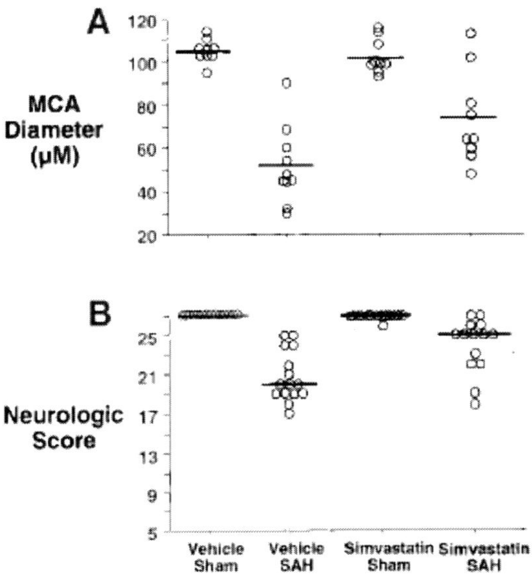

Figure 10. A, MCA lumen diameter 72 hours after SAH or sham surgery in mice treated with vehicle or simvastatin 14 days before SAH or sham surgery and 3 days after surgery. Bars indicate mean values. Circles indicate individual mice. B, Neurological examination scores 72 hours after SAH or sham surgery (27no deficit). Bars indicate median values. Reproduced with permission of Walter Kluwer Health via Copyright Clearance Center's Rights Link (license ID: 3520861185477). Original reference: McGirt, M.J., et al., *Simvastatin Increases Endothelial Nitric Oxide Synthase and Ameliorates Cerebral Vasospasm Resulting From Subarachnoid Hemorrhage*. Stroke, 2002. 33(12): p. 2950-2956. (Figure 2).

A small, prospective, randomized placebo-controlled clinical trial of 80 aSAH patients treated with 40 mg of pravastatin a day against a placebo (for 14 days post-aSAH) showed a significant reduction of severe DV by 42% and a reduction of severe DV by 0.8 days. The incidence of sDV and mortality were significantly decreased by 83% and 75% respectively in the pravastatin group, which supported the findings of the former study [63]. Another small, prospective randomized clinical trial of 39 aSAH patients treated with simvastatin at 80 mg/day against a placebo (for 14 days post-aSAH), showed a safe and significant reduction of DV and TCD mean velocities in the patients treated with simvastatin [64].

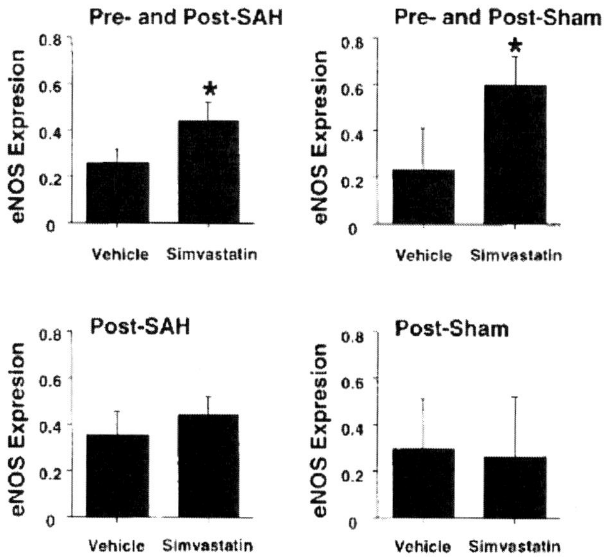

Figure 11. Ipsilateral eNOS protein (pecentage of background optical density) 72 hours after SAH or sham surgery in mice treated with vehicle or simvastatin. Pre- and post- indicates treatment for 14 days before surgery and 3 days after surgery, respectively; Post-, treatment begun after SAH or sham surgery and repeated twice at 24-hour intervals. *P0.05 relative to vehicle-treated cohorts. Values are mean SD. Reproduced with permission of Walter Kluwer Health via Copyright Clearance Center's Rights Link (license ID: 3520861185477). Original reference: McGirt, M.J., et al., *Simvastatin Increases Endothelial Nitric Oxide Synthase and Ameliorates Cerebral Vasospasm Resulting From Subarachnoid Hemorrhage.* Stroke, 2002. 33(12): p. 2950-2956. (Figure 3).

Since then, there have been several retrospective clinical studies, a few small, prospective pilot studies, and, more recently, a prospective multicentre international randomized double–blinded clinical trial (STASH). [65]. The design of these studies and the definition of sDV are heterogeneous Some of the retrospective studies and two small, prospective studies support the use of statins to prevent sDV. STASH enrolled patients were given 40 mg of Simvastatin 96 hours from the ictus for 21 days post–aSAH. The primary outcome of this trial was determined by the distribution of a modified Rankin Scale (mRS) score obtained by questionnaire at 6 months. This trial did not show that statins had any significant effect on the primary outcome measure

[65]. Statin use is still controversial given the contradictory clinical study results. The most important recommendation is to restart the statin therapy if the patient has already been on statins. The rapid withdrawal of statins could exacerbate ischemic cerebrovascular events by causing a rapid reduction of vascular eNOS [51].

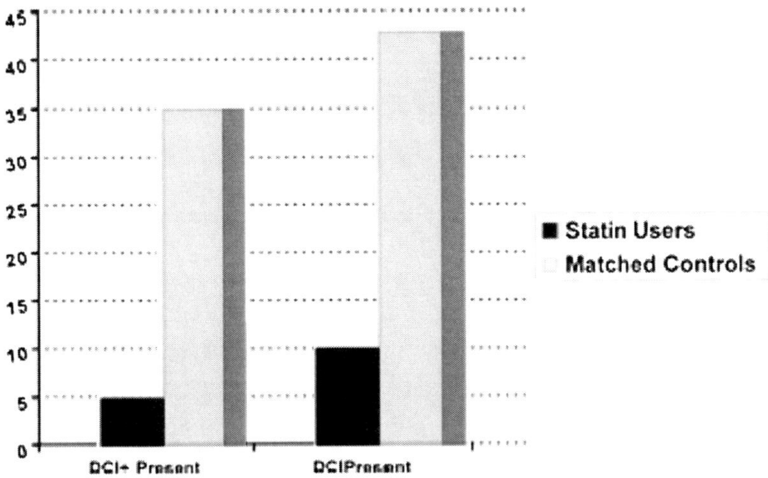

Figure 12. Graph showing comparison of DCI and DCI confirmed by angiogram and/or TCD (DCI) between SAH statin and nonstatin users. A significantly lower incidence of DCI and DCI+ (confirmed with evidence of vasospasm on follow-up angiogram or a TCD-HMV change of 50 cm/s) occurred in the statin group (10% versus 43%, P = 0.02; 5% versus 35%, P = 0.01, respectively) compared with non-statin users. Unpublished original figure from published research). Parra, A., et al., *Effect of prior statin use on functional outcome and delayed vasospasm after acute aneurysmal subarachnoid hemorrhage: a matched controlled cohort study.* Neurosurgery, 2005. 56(3): p. 476-84.

Endovascular Therapy

In the treatment of refractory sDV there have been a myriad of intra-arterial agents and endovascular procedures to vasodilate the affected vessels and prevent permanent ischemic damage in the brain. Intraarterial novocaine, papaverin, and calcium channel blockers have all been administered to patients with refractory sDV.

In 1984, Zubkov et al., reported his experience of using percutaneous endovascular balloon angioplasty of 33 patients with DV. They treated a total of 105 vasospastic arteries and found that patients reported a decrement of focal headache and a regression of focal neurological signs. They reported the improvement of cerebral blood flow (CBF) and electroencephalographic cortical activity for these patients [66]. They also noted that vasoconstriction did not recur in the vessel segments treated with angioplasty, which has been confirmed in other studies as well. The percutaneous endovascular balloon angioplasty of cerebral arteries has not been shown to successfully revert the neurological signs and symptoms of sDV from 31% to 80% [67, 68, 69]. Prospective, randomized clinical trials comparing this therapeutic intervention against placebos or other endovascular therapeutic modalities is lacking. The procedure has some limitations, such as its inability to treat distal segments of the cerebral arteries and its high-risk for complications in patients with atherosclerosis, a profusion of plaque along the walls of tortuous arteries. There have been reports of arterial punctures and dissections, which are serious complications that can result in fatalities and occur in about 5% of cases. This procedure should be reserved for patients who are refractory to medical therapy for sDV.

Papaverine, a phosphodiesterase enzyme inhibitor, has been one of the first intra-arterial agents used for the treatment of refractory sDV. In general, papaverine induces a less marked vasodilation than balloon angioplasty, but the accompanying effects and any observable clinical improvement in the patient are both transient, lasting only a few hours. Many times patients require repeated treatments for sDV. The ensuing complications include, stroke, blindness, increased intracranial pressure, cerebral infarction, and other neurological complications. Some of these complications can be permanent [70]. Because of the short duration of effects and the serious neurological complications associated with it, papaverine has been replaced by other agents, such as calcium channel blockers (e.g. verapamil, nimodipine, and nicardipine) [71, 72, 73] In general, intra-arterial vasodilator infusions are used on patients with distal vasospasm who are unable to undergo treatment with percutaneous balloon angioplasty. It is important to mention that only patients with adequately secured aneurysms can be treated with intra-arterial vasodilators [73]. Calcium channel antagonists and intra-arterial infusions can be used as a single therapy or in conjunction with balloon angioplasty.

A retrospective study of intra-arterial nimodipine for sDV in 25 patients (30 treatments), reported 76% effectiveness in reverting clinical symptoms and 63% visible arterial dilation by angiogram [71]. Badjatia et al., reported their experience administering intra-arterial nicardipine to 18 patients (44 treated arteries) [72]. They observed arterial vasodilation in all the treated arteries and the reversal of neurologic signs and symptoms in 42% of the patients. Furthermore, they reported a significant reduction of TCD mean velocities after the intra-arterial treatments. These patients did not experience any hypotension, but 33% of them developed increased intracranial pressure [10]. The American Heart Association (AHA) considers cerebral angioplasty and/or selective intra-arterial vasodilator therapy to be reasonable treatments for patients with symptomatic cerebral vasospasm, particularly those who are not rapidly responding to hypertensive therapy (Class IIa; Level of Evidence B) [41].

Future Research Directions

Delayed vasospasm is still the most serious complication of aSAH. It negatively impacts the patient's ultimate outcome and has significant costs related to in-hospital monitoring and treatment, as well as post-index hospitalization care.

There is the individual cost of a patient losing his quality of life as well as the social cost of a community losing a productive individual. Vasospasm is still a significant, independent risk factor for poor outcome in patients with aneurysmal SAH [12]. About 50% of the patients who develop sDV die or are left with permanent disability [12]; [10]. These are all important reasons for finding an effective strategy to prevent sDV.

The cascade of events that trigger sDV appear to be multiple in number. Several of them are unleashed almost immediately after the SAH occurs. In order to have a significant protective strategy against DV, clinicians should target the key elements involved in the molecular cascades that lead to DV. Furthermore, clinicians should simultaneously find neuroprotective strategies to use concomitantly with the DV therapy in order to help these patients tolerate ischemia if it occurs.

One area that needs to be investigated further is the microembolic phenomenon associated with VS. A study using aspirin after aneurysmal obliteration in aSAH patients showed it to be safe [25]. Subarachnoid clot drainage is another area worth exploring. The EARLYDRAIN study is ongoing and will evaluate lumbar CSF drainage to prevent sDV [49].

Statins are very attractive to consider for this process because their pleotropic effects have the potential to impact several key targets in the development of DV. It is plausible that, as experimental evidence has demonstrated, the window of action for statins is short. Higher doses of statins could have a more robust effect in modulating the immune response and up-regulating eNOS, but statins do not have homogenous bioavailability or an affinity for lipids, which may affect intracellular signaling effects from these compounds. More clinical research is still needed to answer these questions.

There are newer vasodilator agents and newer routes of delivery to treat sDV. There is a small case series being conducted on calcium channel blockers, sodium nitroprusside, and milrinone given intra-arterially and intrathecally through an external ventricular drain (EVD) or through a lumbar drain (LD) that show promising results. Alternative delivery routes are ideal because they could minimize the systematic effects of vasodilator agents that are problematic for patients at risk of sDV [74, 75, 76, 77].

Finally, there is clinical evidence of an association between the APOE4 allele and a poor outcome after SAH [78]. Dr. Laskowitz and his research team at Duke University developed an APOE-peptide mimetic that has shown neuroprotective effects in a SAH mouse model. This peptide appears to reduce glial activation and central nervous system inflammation after injury [79, 80]. To model the effect of the endogenous APOE genotype on vasospasm and outcome after SAH, they used humanized targeted replacement "knock-in" mice in a clinically relevant model of experimental SAH [78].

These mice only express the human apoE3 or apoE4 protein isoforms at physiological levels in a temporal and spatial pattern similar to the human mechanism. Mice expressing the ApoE4 isoform had greater functional deficit, mortality, cerebral edema, and vasospasm when compared to ApoE3 mice. Mice treated with the APOE-mimetic peptide had decreased mortality, functional deficits, and histological evidence of vasospasm when compared with vehicle-treated animals [78].

Acknowledgments

I would like to thank David Garza, M.A. (Project Coordinator in the Neurosurgery Department at UTHSCSA) for proofreading this manuscript.

References

[1] Pluta, R.M., Delayed cerebral vasospasm and nitric oxide: review, new hypothesis, and proposed treatment. *Pharmacology & Therapeutics*, 2005. 105(1): p. 23-56.

[2] Gull, W., Cases of aneurism of the cerebral vessels. *Guys Hosp. Rep.*, 1859. 5: p. 281-304.

[3] Al-Tamimi, Y.Z., et al., A Review of Delayed Ischemic Neurologic Deficit Following Aneurysmal Subarachnoid Hemorrhage: Historical Overview, Current Treatment, and Pathophysiology. *World Neurosurgery,* 2010. 73(6): p. 654-667.
[4] Sehba, F.A., et al., The importance of early brain injury after subarachnoid hemorrhage. *Progress in neurobiology,* 2012. 97(1): p. 14-37.
[5] Roos, Y., et al., Complications and outcome in patients with aneurysmal subarachnoid hemorrhage: a prospective hospital based cohort study in the Netherlands. Journal of Neurology, *Neurosurgery & Psychiatry,* 2000. 68(3): p. 337-341.
[6] Shimoda, M., et al., Asymptomatic versus symptomatic infarcts from vasospasm in patients with subarachnoid hemorrhage: serial magnetic resonance imaging. *Neurosurgery,* 2001. 49(6): p. 1341-1350.
[7] Brawley, B., D. Strandness Jr, and W. Kelly, The biphasic response of cerebral vasospasm in experimental subarachnoid hemorrhage. *Journal of neurosurgery,* 1968. 28(1): p. 1-8.
[8] Parra, A., et al., Mouse model of subarachnoid hemorrhage associated cerebral vasospasm: methodological analysis. *Neurological research,* 2002. 24(5): p. 510-516.
[9] Rowland, M.J., et al., Delayed cerebral ischaemia after subarachnoid hemorrhage: looking beyond vasospasm. *British Journal of Anaesthesia,* 2012. 109(3): p. 315-329.
[10] Macdonald, R.L., Management of cerebral vasospasm. *Neurosurgical review,* 2006. 29(3): p. 179-193.
[11] Findlay, J.M., et al., A randomized trial of intraoperative, intracisternal tissue plasminogen activator for the prevention of vasospasm. *Neurosurgery,* 1995. 37(1): p. 168-76; discussion 177-8.
[12] Frontera, J.A., et al., Defining Vasospasm After Subarachnoid Hemorrhage What Is the Most Clinically Relevant Definition? *Stroke,* 2009. 40(6): p. 1963-1968.
[13] Khurana, V.G., et al., Update on evidence for a genetic predisposition to cerebral vasospasm. *Neurosurgical Focus,* 2006. 21(3): p. 1-5.
[14] Lanterna, L., et al., APOE influences vasospasm and cognition of noncomatose patients with subarachnoid hemorrhage. *Neurology,* 2005. 64(7): p. 1238-1244.
[15] Oertel, et al., Posttraumatic vasospasm: the epidemiology, severity, and time course of an underestimated phenomenon: a prospective study

performed in 299 patients. *Journal of Neurosurgery,* 2005. 103(5): p. 812-24.

[16] Charpentier, C., et al., Multivariate Analysis of Predictors of Cerebral Vasospasm Occurrence After Aneurysmal Subarachnoid Hemorrhage. *Stroke,* 1999. 30(7): p. 1402-1408.

[17] Claassen, J., et al., Effect of Cisternal and Ventricular Blood on Risk of Delayed Cerebral Ischemia After Subarachnoid Hemorrhage:: The Fisher Scale Revisited. *Stroke,* 2001. 32(9): p. 2012-2020.

[18] Frontera, J.A., et al., Prediction of Symptomatic Vasospasmafter Subarachnoid Hemorrhage: the Modified Fisher Scale. *Neurosurgery,* 2006. 59(1): p. 21-27.

[19] Mayberg, M.R., T. Okada, and D.H. Bark, The role of hemoglobin in arterial narrowing after subarachnoid hemorrhage. *Journal of Neurosurgery,* 1990. 72(4): p. 634-640.

[20] Chokyu, M., An experimental study of cerebral vasospasm, especially on spasmogenic factors in red blood cells. *Osaka City Med. J.,* 1975. 24: p. 211-221.

[21] Ding, D., et al., Therapeutic implications of estrogen for cerebral vasospasm and delayed cerebral ischemia induced by aneurysmal subarachnoid hemorrhage. *BioMed research international,* 2014. 2014.

[22] McGirt, M.J., et al., Attenuation of Cerebral Vasospasm After Subarachnoid Hemorrhage in Mice Overexpressing Extracellular Superoxide Dismutase. *Stroke,* 2002. 33(9): p. 2317-2323.

[23] Eich, R.F., et al., Mechanism of NO-induced oxidation of myoglobin and hemoglobin. *Biochemistry,* 1996. 35(22): p. 6976-6983.

[24] Borsody, M., et al., Haptoglobin and the development of cerebral artery vasospasm after subarachnoid hemorrhage. *Neurology,* 2006. 66(5): p. 634-640.

[25] Hop, J., et al., Randomized pilot trial of postoperative aspirin in subarachnoid hemorrhage. *Neurology,* 2000. 54(4): p. 872-878.

[26] Borel, C.O., et al., Possible Role for Vascular Cell Proliferation in Cerebral Vasospasm After Subarachnoid Hemorrhage. *Stroke,* 2003. 34(2): p. 427-433.

[27] Romano, J.G., et al., Detection of microemboli by transcranial Doppler ultrasonography in aneurysmal subarachnoid hemorrhage. *Neurosurgery,* 2002. 50(5): p. 1026-1031.

[28] Zimmermann, M. and V. Seifert, Endothelin receptor antagonists and cerebral vasospasm. *Clinical Autonomic Research,* 2004. 14(3): p. 143-145.

[29] Carr, K.R., S.L. Zuckerman, and J. Mocco, Inflammation, Cerebral Vasospasm, and Evolving Theories of Delayed Cerebral Ischemia. *Neurology Research International,* 2013. 2013: p. 12.
[30] Osuka, K., et al., Interleukin-6 and development of vasospasm after subarachnoid hemorrhage. *Acta neurochirurgica,* 1998. 140(9): p. 943-951.
[31] Lim, M., et al., The predictive value of serum myeloperoxidase for vasospasm in patients with aneurysmal subarachnoid hemorrhage. *Neurosurgical review,* 2012. 35(3): p. 413-419.
[32] Bowman, G., et al., Neutralizing antibody against interleukin-6 attenuates posthemorrhagic vasospasm in the rat femoral artery model. *Neurosurgery,* 2004. 54(3): p. 719-726.
[33] Aihara, Y., et al., Quantitative analysis of gene expressions related to inflammation in canine spastic artery after subarachnoid hemorrhage. *Stroke,* 2001. 32(1): p. 212-217.
[34] Vecchione, C., et al., Tumor Necrosis Factor-α Mediates Hemolysis-Induced Vasoconstriction and the Cerebral Vasospasm Evoked by Subarachnoid Hemorrhage. *Hypertension,* 2009. 54(1): p. 150-156.
[35] Leao, A., Spreading depression of activity in the cerebral cortex, 1943, *Am. Physiological. Soc.,*
[36] Temes, R.E., et al., Left ventricular dysfunction and cerebral infarction from vasospasm after subarachnoid hemorrhage. *Neurocritical care,* 2010. 13(3): p. 359-365.
[37] Wartenberg, K.E., et al., Acute ischemic injury on diffusion-weighted magnetic resonance imaging after poor grade subarachnoid hemorrhage. *Neurocritical care,* 2011. 14(3): p. 407-415.
[38] De Marchis, G., et al., Brain Injury Visible on Early MRI After Subarachnoid Hemorrhage Might Predict Neurological Impairment and Functional Outcome. *Neurocritical Care,* 2014: p. 1-8.
[39] Van den Bergh, W., et al., Magnetic resonance imaging in experimental subarachnoid hemorrhage. *Acta Neurochirurgica,* 2005. 147(9): p. 977-983.
[40] Dorsch, N. and M. King, A review of cerebral vasospasm in aneurysmal subarachnoid hemorrhage Part I: Incidence and effects. *Journal of Clinical Neuroscience,* 1994. 1(1): p. 19-26.
[41] Connolly, E.S., et al., Guidelines for the management of aneurysmal subarachnoid hemorrhage a guideline for healthcare professionals from the American heart association/American stroke association. *Stroke,* 2012. 43(6): p. 1711-1737.

[42] Sloan, M., et al., Sensitivity and specificity of transcranial Doppler ultrasonography in the diagnosis of vasospasm following subarachnoid hemorrhage. *Neurology,* 1989. 39(11): p. 1514-1514.

[43] Nosko, M., et al., Effect of clot removal at 24 hours on chronic vasospasm after SAH in the primate model. *Journal of neurosurgery,* 1987. 66(3): p. 416-422.

[44] Mizukami, M., et al., Prevention of vasospasm by early operation with removal of subarachnoid blood. *Neurosurgery,* 1982. 10(3): p. 301-307.

[45] Findlay, J., et al., The effect of timing of intrathecal fibrinolytic therapy on cerebral vasospasm in a primate model of subarachnoid hemorrhage. *Neurosurgery,* 1990. 26(2): p. 201-206.

[46] Seifert, V., et al., Prevention of delayed ischaemic deficits after aneurysmal subarachnoid hemorrhage by intrathecal bolus injection of tissue plasminogen activator (rTPA). *Acta neurochirurgica,* 1994. 128(1-4): p. 137-143.

[47] Hamada, J.-i., et al., Effect on Cerebral Vasospasm of Coil Embolization Followed by Microcatheter Intrathecal Urokinase Infusion Into the Cisterna Magna A Prospective Randomized Study. *Stroke,* 2003. 34(11): p. 2549-2554.

[48] Al-Tamimi, Y.Z., et al., Lumbar Drainage of Cerebrospinal Fluid After Aneurysmal Subarachnoid Hemorrhage A Prospective, Randomized, Controlled Trial (LUMAS). *Stroke,* 2012. 43(3): p. 677-682.

[49] Bardutzky, J., et al., EARLYDRAIN-outcome after early lumbar CSF-drainage in aneurysmal subarachnoid hemorrhage: study protocol for a randomized controlled trial. *Trials,* 2011. 12(1): p. 203.

[50] Lennihan, L., et al., Effect of Hypervolemic Therapy on Cerebral Blood Flow After Subarachnoid Hemorrhage: A Randomized Controlled Trial. *Stroke,* 2000. 31(2): p. 383-391.

[51] Diringer, M.N., et al., Critical care management of patients following aneurysmal subarachnoid hemorrhage: recommendations from the Neurocritical Care Society's Multidisciplinary Consensus Conference. *Neurocritical care,* 2011. 15(2): p. 211-240.

[52] Barker, F.G. and C.S. Ogilvy, Efficacy of prophylactic nimodipine for delayed ischemic deficit after subarachnoid hemorrhage: a metaanalysis. *Journal of neurosurgery*, 1996. 84(3): p. 405-414.

[53] Dorsch, N., N. Kassell, and M. Sinkula, Metaanalysis of trials of tirilazad mesylate in aneurysmal SAH. Acta neurochirurgica. *Supplement,* 2001. 77: p. 233.

[54] Sauzeau, V., et al., Cyclic GMP-dependent protein kinase signaling pathway inhibits RhoA-induced Ca2+ sensitization of contraction in vascular smooth muscle. *Journal of Biological Chemistry,* 2000. 275 (28): p. 21722-21729.

[55] Shibuya, M., et al., Effect of AT877 on cerebral vasospasm after aneurysmal subarachnoid hemorrhage: results of a prospective placebo-controlled double-blind trial. *Journal of neurosurgery,* 1992. 76(4): p. 571-577.

[56] Vajkoczy, P., et al., Clazosentan (AXV-034343), a selective endothelin A receptor antagonist, in the prevention of cerebral vasospasm following severe aneurysmal subarachnoid hemorrhage: results of a randomized, double-blind, placebo-controlled, multicenter Phase IIa study. *Journal of Neurosurgery,* 2005. 103(1): p. 9-17.

[57] Macdonald, R.L., et al., Randomized Trial of Clazosentan in Patients With Aneurysmal Subarachnoid Hemorrhage Undergoing Endovascular Coiling. *Stroke,* 2012. 43(6): p. 1463-1469.

[58] Sadeh, M., Action of magnesium sulfate in the treatment of preeclampsia-eclampsia. *Stroke,* 1989. 20(9): p. 1273-5.

[59] Marinov, M.B., et al., Neuroprotective effects of preischemia intraarterial magnesium sulfate in reversible focal cerebral ischemia. *Journal of neurosurgery,* 1996. 85(1): p. 117-124.

[60] Wong, G.K.C., et al., Intravenous magnesium sulphate for aneurysmal subarachnoid hemorrhage (IMASH) a randomized, double-blinded, placebo-controlled, multicenter phase III trial. *Stroke,* 2010. 41(5): p. 921-926.

[61] McGirt, M.J., et al., Simvastatin Increases Endothelial Nitric Oxide Synthase and Ameliorates Cerebral Vasospasm Resulting From Subarachnoid Hemorrhage. *Stroke,* 2002. 33(12): p. 2950-2956.

[62] Parra, A., et al., Effect of prior statin use on functional outcome and delayed vasospasm after acute aneurysmal subarachnoid hemorrhage: a matched controlled cohort study. *Neurosurgery,* 2005. 56(3): p. 476-84; discussion 476-84.

[63] Tseng, M.-Y., et al., Effects of Acute Treatment With Pravastatin on Cerebral Vasospasm, Autoregulation, and Delayed Ischemic Deficits After Aneurysmal Subarachnoid Hemorrhage A Phase II Randomized Placebo-Controlled Trial. *Stroke,* 2005. 36(8): p. 1627-1632.

[64] Lynch, J.R., et al., Simvastatin reduces vasospasm after aneurysmal subarachnoid hemorrhage results of a pilot randomized clinical trial. *Stroke,* 2005. 36(9): p. 2024-2026.

[65] Kirkpatrick, P.J., et al., Simvastatin in aneurysmal subarachnoid hemorrhage (STASH): a multicentre randomised phase 3 trial. *The Lancet Neurology,* 2014. 13(7): p. 666-675.
[66] Zubkov, A.Y., et al., Mechanism of Endothelin-1–Induced Contraction in Rabbit Basilar Artery. *Stroke,* 2000. 31(2): p. 526-533.
[67] Bejjani, G.K., et al., The efficacy and safety of angioplasty for cerebral vasospasm after subarachnoid hemorrhage. *Neurosurgery,* 1998. 42(5): p. 979-986.
[68] Coyne, T., et al., Percutaneous transluminal angioplasty for cerebral vasospasm after subarachnoid hemorrhage. Canadian journal of surgery. *Journal canadien de chirurgie,* 1994. 37(5): p. 391-396.
[69] Eskridge, J., D. Newell, and G. Pendleton, Transluminal angioplasty for treatment of vasospasm. *Neurosurgery clinics of North America,* 1990. 1(2): p. 387-399.
[70] Smith, W.S., et al., Neurotoxicity of intra-arterial papaverine preserved with chlorobutanol used for the treatment of cerebral vasospasm after aneurysmal subarachnoid hemorrhage. *Stroke,* 2004. 35(11): p. 2518-2522.
[71] Biondi, A., et al., Intra-Arterial Nimodipine for the Treatment of Symptomatic Cerebral Vasospasm after Aneurysmal Subarachnoid Hemorrhage: Preliminary Results. *American Journal of Neuroradiology,* 2004. 25(6): p. 1067-1076.
[72] Badjatia, N., et al., Preliminary experience with intra-arterial nicardipine as a treatment for cerebral vasospasm. *American journal of neuroradiology,* 2004. 25(5): p. 819-826.
[73] Macdonald, R.L., Cerebral vasospasm. *Neurosurgery Quarterly,* 1995. 5(2): p. 73-97.
[74] Zhang, Y.P., et al., Intrathecal Treatment of Cerebral Vasospasm. *Journal of Stroke and Cerebrovascular Diseases,* 2013. 22(8): p. 1201-1211.
[75] Sadamasa, N., et al., Milrinone Via Lumbar Subarachnoid Catheter for Vasospasm After Aneurysmal Subarachnoid Hemorrhage. *Neurocritical Care,* 2014: p. 1-6.
[76] Shankar, J.J.S., et al., Angiographic evaluation of the effect of intra-arterial milrinone therapy in patients with vasospasm from aneurysmal subarachnoid hemorrhage. *Neuroradiology,* 2011. 53(2): p. 123-128.
[77] Thomas, J.E., et al., Safety of intrathecal sodium nitroprusside for the treatment and prevention of refractory cerebral vasospasm and ischemia in humans. *Stroke,* 1999. 30(7): p. 1409-1416.

[78] Gao, J., et al., A novel apoE-derived therapeutic reduces vasospasm and improves outcome in a murine model of subarachnoid hemorrhage. *Neurocritical Care,* 2006. 4(1): p. 25-31.

[79] Laskowitz, D., et al., Apolipoprotein E suppresses glial cell secretion of TNF< i> α</i>. *Journal of neuroimmunology,* 1997. 76(1): p. 70-74.

[80] Laskowitz, D., et al., Downregulation of microglial activation by apolipoprotein E and apoE-mimetic peptides. *Experimental neurology,* 2001. 167(1): p. 74-85.

In: Subarachnoid Hemorrhage
Editor: Linda R. Gray
ISBN: 978-1-63463-492-2

Chapter 2

Hydrocephalus Following Spontaneous Subarachnoid Hemorrhage: Its Occurrence and Implications

Marguerite A. Butchee[1], Bradley N. Bohnstedt[2] and Bappaditya Ray[1*]
[1]Department of Neurology and
[2]Department of Neurological Surgery
The University of Oklahoma Health Sciences Center,
Oklahoma City, Oklahoma, US

Abstract

Hydrocephalus is a common complication after spontaneous subarachnoid hemorrhage (SAH). It is seen in 15-20% of acute (48-72 hours), 2-3% of subacute (4-13 days) and 10-20% of chronic (after 14 days) cases.

* *Communicating author:* Bappaditya Ray, MBBS, MD, Division of Critical Care Neurology, Department of Neurology, 920 Stanton L Young Blvd; Ste 2040, Oklahoma City, OK 73104, Phone - +1-405-271-4113, Fax - +1-405-271-5763; e-mail: Bappaditya-Ray@ouhsc.edu

SAH patients presenting with poor neurological status and presence of hydrocephalus are known indicators for adverse outcome. Although the exact mechanism for hydrocephalus remains ill-defined, leading theories include obstruction of cerebrospinal fluid (CSF) flow through the ventricles and compromised CSF reabsorption through the arachnoid granulations due to its obstruction by blood products. More recent theories propose fibrosis leading to obstruction of the fourth ventricle and arachnoid granulations, and also increased CSF production resulting in hydrocephalus. Acute hydrocephalus following SAH is usually managed by temporary CSF diversion using external ventricular drain (EVD) or lumbar drain. There are several advantages and disadvantages of the above-mentioned procedures and its placement is determined usually by patient specific issues and local practice. Above-mentioned temporary diversion procedures are gradually weaned over a period of days with the goal of discontinuation once the CSF flow dynamics have normalized. Unfortunately, guidelines are lacking regarding such weaning protocols. The number of patients who undergo permanent CSF diversion procedure is variable depending of neurosurgeons' preference that maybe based on radiological evidence of hydrocephalus versus symptomatic hydrocephalus.

Introduction

The term hydrocephalus of derived from Greek words – *'hydros'* meaning water and *'cephalus'* meaning head. It is one of the common complications after spontaneous subarachnoid hemorrhage (SAH). Hydrocephalus can occur at different stages of this disease process – acutely (0-3 days), subacutely (4-13 days) or chronically (≥ 14 days). Exact mechanism for development of this complication after SAH is unknown, though various theories have been postulated.

The radiological features may or may not have clinical correlation. This may be attributed to inter-individual variation in compensatory reserve of their brain microenvironmental physiology. In other words, how much a brain can adapt to the altered milieu secondary to hydrocephalus. Initial and final management of this complication varies among different centers and mostly guided by local expertise and some retrospective case series. In this review our aim is to bring forward inherent problems associated with hydrocephalus following SAH, discuss its pathophysiology for better understanding of its symptomatology and thus facilitate development of standardized management strategies for this debilitating neurological condition after SAH.

Epidemiology

The incidence of hydrocephalus after SAH is varied. Reported incidence of acute hydrocephalus needing external ventricular drainage (EVD) during the acute phase of illness is 26-47% [1-4]. Although, its incidence after SAH is frequently quoted as 6-67% [1, 5]. Variation in number is most likely related to difference in criteria used to determine its occurrence and physician's interpretation. Radiological criteria may overestimate while clinical criteria may underestimate the incidence [6]. A review of 3521 cases of SAH in the Co-operative Aneurysm Study demonstrated clinically symptomatic hydrocephalus in 13.3% [5]. Acute hydrocephalus (radiological) was present in 9.1% of patients, with delayed (clinical) was present in 7.3% and there was 6% overlap. Local clinical practice may also contribute to varying EVD requirement after SAH. In a study of 108 patients with SAH, 10% of patients required EVD placement before intervention for their clinical condition while 80% ended up with cerebrospinal fluid (CSF) diversion after surgery [7]. Similar variations are also noted in permanent CSF diversion with reported incidence of 6.5-25% [1-3, 8, 9].

Various clinical and radiological parameters are identified as predictors of acute and chronic hydrocephalus requiring ventriculoperitoneal (VP) shunt placement. The most common variables for acute symptomatic hydrocephalus in order of importance are: hydrocephalus demonstrated on CT head, intraventricular hemorrhage (IVH), level of consciousness at admission, increasing age, amount of subarachnoid blood, posterior circulation site and post-operative hypertension [5, 10]. Similarly, several predisposing factors like women, increasing age, poor admission neurological grade, IVH, acute hydrocephalus, meningitis, vasospasm, aneurysm location and endovascular treatment have been recognized as important contributors to the development of chronic hydrocephalus [1, 5, 7, 8, 11, 12].

Pathophysiology of Hydrocephalus after Subarachnoid Hemorrhage

According to the classical theory of CSF circulation (bulk flow theory), CSF is primarily synthesized in the choroid plexus of the lateral ventricles and flows through successive ventricles and then into the subarachnoid space and eventually reabsorbed in the arachnoid granulations located in the superior sagittal sinus (Figure 1). The classical theory has been challenged by recently described alternate theory of CSF formation and circulation (based on CSF hydrodynamics) that hypothesizes that the interstitial fluid (ISF) and CSF constitute a functional unit and are regulated by changes in osmotic and hydrostatic pressure in central nervous system (CNS) microvessels (Figure 2) [13]. There is continuous turnover of ISF–CSF bulk that is created by the filtration of water across arterial capillary walls under hydrostatic pressure and the reabsorption of water from the interstitium into the venous capillaries and postcapillary venules by osmotic counter-pressure. Circulation of CSF is also dependent on arterial pulsation transmitted in the cranium as demonstrated by magnetic resonance imaging (MRI) studies [14-16]. During systole, the flow of additional blood into the rigid cranium forces a volume of intracranial CSF out through the foramen magnum (in order to maintain constant volume as per Kellie-Monroe hypothesis) and then the mesencephalic aqueduct. During diastole, venous draining causes a drop in pressure in the cranium and enables CSF to flow back into the cranium from the spinal channel via the foramen magnum and the mesencephalic aqueduct. Hence, during a cardiac cycle, the CSF pulsates through the mesencephalic aqueduct and the foramen magnum during normal physiologic CSF circulation.

The leading theory of acute hydrocephalus after SAH, hypothesize clogging of leptomeninges and arachnoid granulations with blood breakdown products and fibrin and thus resulting in impairment of CSF flow and absorption [17]. This process may subsequently result in fibrosis of the above-mentioned structures and cause chronic hydrocephalus development. Credence to the acute obstructive hydrocephalus theory is most likely supported by increased incidence of hydrocephalus associated with posterior circulation aneurysm ruptures, leading to obstruction in CSF egress from fourth ventricle into the subarachnoid space [5, 17]. On the contrary, it is postulated that anterior circulation aneurysmal rupture cause hydrocephalus primarily by fibrosis of the leptomeninges and arachnoid granulations and result in a communicating pattern of hydrocephalus in the acute and chronic states [17]. However, treatment modalities like third ventriculostomy and lamina terminalis fenestration have resulted in decreased incidence of VP shunt [17, 18] allude to other factors contributing to development of acute hydrocephalus. Alternate theory of CSF circulation including hydrodynamic theory can better explain the occurrence of hydrocephalus following SAH. Presence of blood in the subarachnoid space causes an acute rise in CSF osmolarity and/or hydrostatic pressure after aneurysm rupture.

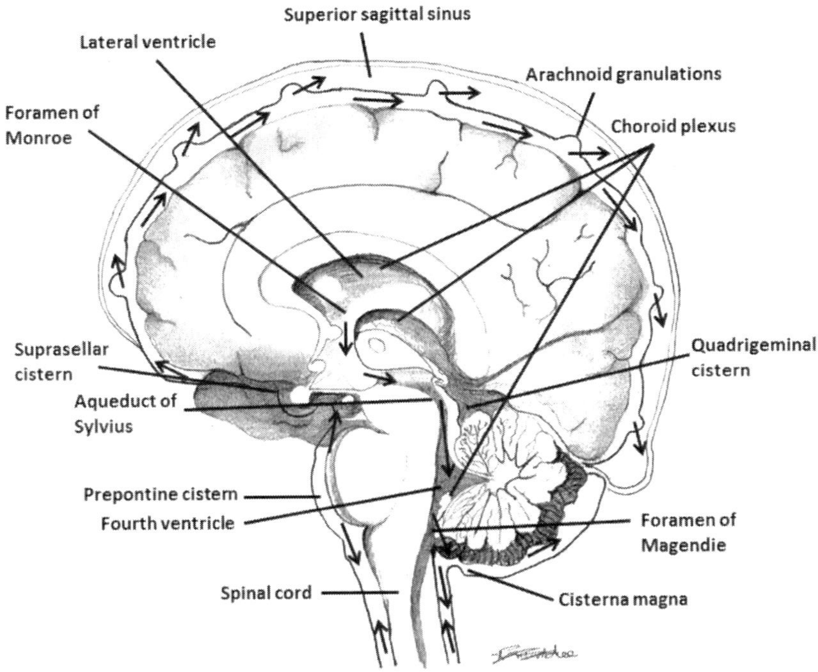

Figure 1. Classical theory of cerebrospinal fluid (CSF) circulation. Schematic diagram of mid-sagittal section of human brain shows production of CSF from the choroid plexus and its circulation through the ventricular system and egress into the subarachnoid space through median aperture, Foramen of Magendie and lateral apertures, foramina of Lushka (not depicted). The CSF subsequently flows into the spinal subarachnoid space and returns back to the cranium during cardiac diastole to be absorbed in the venous sinuses via arachnoid granulations.

This leads to increased CSF production through transcapillary water transport from the cerebral microvasculature. Such increased CSF production with increase in CSF osmolarity has been demonstrated in feline models of hydrocephalus [19, 20]. Moreover, increased numbers of water vesicles were noted during the acute phase in the choroid plexus of rabbits with SAH [21]. Authors postulated stimulation of glossopharyngeal and vagus nerves in increased production of CSF from choroid plexus. Presence of IVH in SAH is also frequently associated with acute hydrocephalus and is postulated to be due to obstruction at the level of cerebral aqueduct. But a CSF flow study using MRI techniques did not show decreased flow at the level of cerebral aqueduct as may expected in SAH patient with intraventricular hemorrhage [16]. Increased or normal flows were noted in these patients with acute hydrocephalus after SAH. Thus substantiating increased CSF production and/or decreased CSF resorption and possible absence of CSF outflow obstruction as that would have caused decreased CSF flow.

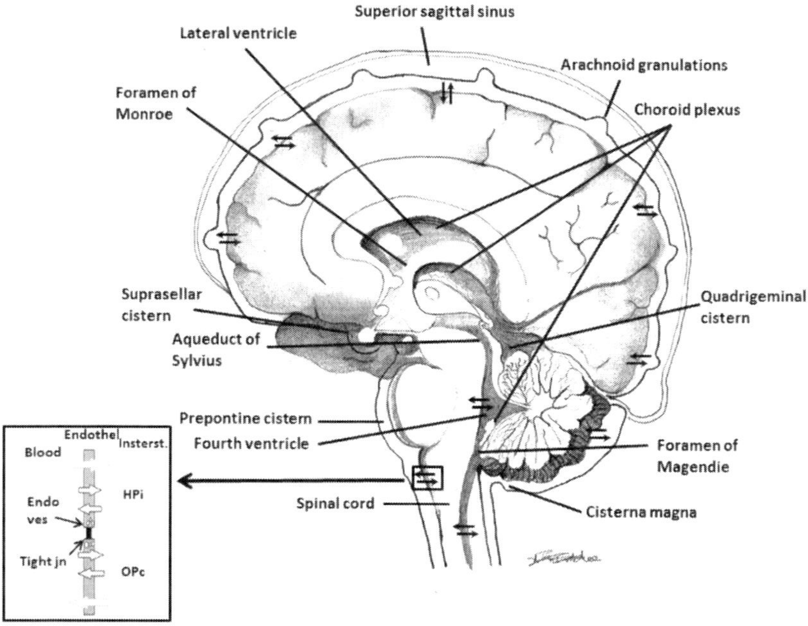

Figure 2. Alternate theory of cerebrospinal fluid (CSF) circulation. Schematic diagram of mid-sagittal section of human brain shows production of CSF through trans-capillary filtration as indicated by the bi-directional arrows. The basic principle is elaborated in the insert diagram showing direction of flow of CSF is dependent on interstitial hydrostatic pressure (HPi) and intercellular osmotic pressure (OPc). Enodhel – endothelium; Endo. ves. – Endocytic vesicles; Interst – Interstitium; Tight jn. – Tight junction.

The cause of chronic hydrocephalus is more complex and poorly understood [10, 17]. It is unlikely that increased CSF production is responsible for such hydrocephalus as it has been demonstrated in animal model that there is atrophy of choroid plexus during late phase of SAH [21]. Clinical associations of shunt dependent hydrocephalus in elderly patients, presence of cerebral infarction, meningitis/ ventriculitis most likely indicate alteration in cerebral compliance with decreased brain elasticity. It would be difficult to explain ventricular enlargement causing hydrocephalus in the chronic phase after SAH.

In such an event there should be enlargement in the subarachnoid space and not the ventricular system. This phenomenon is demonstrated in kaolin-induced communicating hydrocephalus model and explained by redistribution of CSF pulsation in the cranium [13, 22]. Hence, most likely there is higher ventricular system pulsation and lower subarachnoid space pulsations in the chronic phase after SAH leading to development of shunt dependent hydrocephalus.

To summarize, pathophysiology of hydrocephalus after SAH is complex and multifactorial. During the acute phase it is most likely due to CSF flow obstruction and CSF overproduction with minimal contribution from decreased CSF reabsorption. In contrast, chronic hydrocephalus is most likely related to structural changes in the CSF circulation and brain microenvironment leading to qualitative differential transmantle pressure gradient.

Clinical Manifestations and Diagnosis

Most common presentation in patients with SAH is headache, nausea and vomiting. Hydrocephalus may contribute to the headache component due to its pressure effect on pain-sensitive meningeal structures. Other commonly associated symptom with hydrocephalus is alteration in consciousness or lethargy and most likely is due to its effect on ascending reticular activating system and its thalamocortical projections. Enlargement of the bilateral lateral ventricles would cause bicortical dysfunction while pathological increase in third ventricle would affect thalamic function. Impaired upgaze maybe pathognomonic of hydrocephalus and is due to dysfunction of the dorsal midbrain vertical gaze center.

There are several ventricular measurement techniques established for CT related diagnosis of hydrocephalus. Most commonly used marker is bicaudate index. It is calculated by drawing a line between the maximum width of the lateral ventricles at the level of caudate nuclei divided by the corresponding diameter of the line connecting the inner table of the skull at the same level. Using control data from 2 separate groups of patients without neurological disease and showing the distribution of bicaudate values, van Gijn and colleagues proposed that hydrocephalus should be diagnosed when the bicaudate index was more than the age-corrected 95th percentile [23].

Treatment

Acute and/or Temporary CSF Diversion

External Ventricular Drain

External ventricular drains (EVDs) have traditionally been used in acute setting for CSF drainage after SAH. It also allows for measuring and monitoring of intracranial pressure. Most commonly, it is placed frontally at Kocher's point with the tip of the catheter being placed within the foramen of Monroe [24]. At times, CSF drainage is needed for cerebral relaxation intraoperatively and requires ventricular access via an EVD at perisylvian region, Paine's point [25]. The EVD placement is beneficial for drainage of CSF from the ventricle, intracranial pressure monitoring and facilitating clearing of intraventricular blood. Unfortunately, EVDs are associated with several complications. These include hemorrhage (1-32%) [26, 27], malposition (6-20%), infection rate (4-10%) depending on duration of placement, with daily rate of up to 10.3% following day 6 of insertion [26, 28, 29], blockage (~6%) [28], and permanent neurological injury of ~1% [30].

Lumbar Cisternal Drainage

Another point of access to the subarachnoid space is the lumbar cistern. A catheter can be placed in this space for drainage of CSF through serial lumbar punctures [31]. A study from England suggested that lumbar drainage, as opposed to ventricular drainage, may provide an additional benefit of reducing vasospasm [32]. Access to the lumbar subarachnoid cistern has potential complications of epidural/subdural hematoma, abscess, meningitis, over drainage associated intracranial hypotension and headache (2-59%) [33, 34], nerve root injury, and retained catheter with removal (5-13%) [31, 34-36]. Although rare, significant over-drainage from an unattended lumbar drain can cause cerebellar herniation [34, 37]. Hence, caution needs to be exercised while using this modality for temporary CSF diversion and this would need additional nursing training and developing familiarity with this drainage procedure.

Fenestration of Lamina Terminalis

During surgical clip ligation of aneurysms where the optic chiasm and lamina terminalis is explored, fenestration of the lamina terminalis can be performed allowing egress of CSF into the subarachnoid space [38]. This is particularly advantageous when there is significant third ventricular hemorrhage. It does not infrequently aid in reducing subsequent need for external ventricular drain if not already placed for obstructive hydrocephalus and brain relaxation during craniotomy. Some reports claim lamina terminalis fenestration reduces permanent CSF diversion rates to 2.3% [18]. But recent meta-analysis did not show clinically significant difference in developing shunt-dependent hydrocephalus with 10% in lamina terminalis fenestration group and 14% in non-interventional group ($p = 0.089$) requiring permanent CSF diversion [39].

Third Ventriculostomy

When hydrocephalus is associated with obstruction due to IVH associated with SAH, endoscopic third ventriculostomy (ETV) is a surgical option to facilitate bypassing of CSF into the subarachnoid space. A retrospective single center study reported rates of permanent CSF diversion with such implantable devices may be reduced by up to 80 percent [40]. However, if ETV is performed in a delayed fashion (~30 days) for symptomatic hydrocephalus there may be temporary improvement in cognitive functioning but its effect it not sustained with 5 out of 8 patients eventually needing permanent CSF diversion [41].

Chronic and/or Permanent CSF Diversion

Cerebral Ventricular Drainage Shunt

When a patient cannot be weaned from their temporary CSF diversion, the most common choice of permanent diversion is with a ventriculoperiotoneal (VP) shunts. Rapid and gradual wean has been analyzed in a single center study in a randomized design but did not show any difference in permanent shunt requirement [42]. Another single center study analyzed continuous CSF drainage against intermittent CSF drainage as per predetermined intracranial pressure threshold [43]. Though there was no difference in determination of permanent CSF diversion, this study showed increased EVD related complications – as defined as non-patent EVD, ventriculitis and CSF leak/hemorrhage in the continuous CSF drainage group. When permanent shunt requirement is determined, a ventricular catheter is either placed similarly to that of an external ventricular drain or parieto-occipitally at Frazier's point [44]. A single center case series did not show any increased rate of infection or shunt failures when the EVD entrance site was used to convert it to VP shunt [45]. Moreover, in this study there was no role of increased protein or red blood cell count in determination of shunt failure. Whichever access point is determined for shunt placement, the ventricular catheter is attached to a reservoir for percutaneous access and a valve for regulation of CSF flow. Valves may be fixed in pressure or programmable which may require confirmation of setting after magnetic resonance imaging studies. Occasionally, shunt assistants of anti-siphon devices are required to help further regulate flow in relation to position of the patient. The valve is then connected to a distal catheter that is commonly placed in the peritoneum. Alternative locations for distal catheter placement include the right atrium of the heart [46], the pleura [47], and the gall bladder [48].

Lumboperitoneal Shunt

The lumboperitoneal shunt uses a catheter that accesses the lumbar cistern and then is passed subcutaneously and drained into the peritoneum via a sialastic tube with slit valves on the peritoneal side. Valves that regulate this flow do exist, but are less commonly used. Once a shunt is placed, a patient typically becomes dependent on the CSF diversion provided by it. If the flow through the drainage system is reduced or obstructed, a revision may be required to restore flow. Symptoms suggesting reduced or obstructed flow include increased lethargy, positional headaches, headaches upon awakening, abducens nerve palsies, unexplained nausea and vomiting, gait instability, and new urinary incontinence. A single center case series suggested poor clinical outcome in patients undergoing lumboperitoneal shunting as compared to VP shunt placement [49]. But previous series had shown better efficacy and lower shunt revision rates of 16% in SAH population as compared to VP shunt [50].

Conclusion

Many questions pertaining to the development and management of hydrocephalus after SAH remain unanswered. Determination of pathophysiology of hydrocephalus after SAH would require concerted effort between clinicians and basic scientists to determine its etiology. From treatment perspective, conducting a systematic randomized trial in this subpopulation of SAH patients may be difficult. The available literature (although mostly retrospective and case series) recommends temporary CSF diversion in cases of symptomatic hydrocephalus and eventual permanent shunting using various procedures. There is no definite guideline or systematic criteria to predict permanent shunt diversion. There remains a need for better studies to delineate predictors for shunt requirement in order to decrease length of hospital stay and also on methodology in determination of permanent CSF diversion.

References

[1] Dorai Z, Hynan LS, Kopitnik TA, Samson D: Factors related to hydrocephalus after aneurysmal subarachnoid hemorrhage. *Neurosurgery* 2003, 52(4):763-769; discussion 769-771.

[2] Yang TC, Chang CH, Liu YT, Chen YL, Tu PH, Chen HC: Predictors of shunt-dependent chronic hydrocephalus after aneurysmal subarachnoid hemorrhage. *European neurology* 2013, 69(5):296-303.

[3] Rincon F, Gordon E, Starke RM, Buitrago MM, Fernandez A, Schmidt JM, Claassen J, Wartenberg KE, Frontera J, Seder DB *et al*: Predictors of long-term shunt-dependent hydrocephalus after aneurysmal subarachnoid hemorrhage. Clinical article. *Journal of neurosurgery* 2010, 113(4):774-780.

[4] Mehta V, Holness RO, Connolly K, Walling S, Hall R: Acute hydrocephalus following aneurysmal subarachnoid hemorrhage. *Can. J. Neurol. Sci.* 1996, 23(1):40-45.

[5] Graff-Radford NR, Torner J, Adams HP, Jr., Kassell NF: Factors associated with hydrocephalus after subarachnoid hemorrhage. A report of the Cooperative Aneurysm Study. *Arch. Neurol.* 1989, 46(7):744-752.

[6] Hasan D, Vermeulen M, Wijdicks EF, Hijdra A, van Gijn J: Management problems in acute hydrocephalus after subarachnoid hemorrhage. *Stroke; a journal of cerebral circulation* 1989, 20(6):747-753.

[7] Vale FL, Bradley EL, Fisher WS, 3rd: The relationship of subarachnoid hemorrhage and the need for postoperative shunting. *Journal of neurosurgery* 1997, 86(3):462-466.

[8] Lai L, Morgan MK: Predictors of in-hospital shunt-dependent hydrocephalus following rupture of cerebral aneurysms. *Journal of clinical neuroscience : official journal of the Neurosurgical Society of Australasia* 2013, 20(8):1134-1138.

[9] O'Kelly CJ, Kulkarni AV, Austin PC, Urbach D, Wallace MC: Shunt-dependent hydrocephalus after aneurysmal subarachnoid hemorrhage:

incidence, predictors, and revision rates. Clinical article. *Journal of neurosurgery* 2009, 111(5):1029-1035.

[10] McCormick PW: Elevated Intracranial Pressure, Ventricular Drainage, and Hydrocephalus after Subarachnoid Hemorrhage. In: *Subarachnoid Hemorrhage: Pathophysiology and Management.* Edited by Bederson JB. Park Ridge, IL: The American Association of Neurological Surgeons; 1997: 77-88.

[11] Kwon JH, Sung SK, Song YJ, Choi HJ, Huh JT, Kim HD: Predisposing factors related to shunt-dependent chronic hydrocephalus after aneurysmal subarachnoid hemorrhage. *Journal of Korean Neurosurgical Society* 2008, 43(4):177-181.

[12] Tapaninaho A, Hernesniemi J, Vapalahti M, Niskanen M, Kari A, Luukkonen M, Puranen M: Shunt-dependent hydrocephalus after subarachnoid hemorrhage and aneurysm surgery: timing of surgery is not a risk factor. *Acta Neurochir (Wien)* 1993, 123(3-4):118-124.

[13] Oreskovic D, Klarica M: Development of hydrocephalus and classical hypothesis of cerebrospinal fluid hydrodynamics: facts and illusions. *Prog Neurobiol* 2011, 94(3):238-258.

[14] Baledent O, Henry-Feugeas MC, Idy-Peretti I: Cerebrospinal fluid dynamics and relation with blood flow: a magnetic resonance study with semiautomated cerebrospinal fluid segmentation. *Invest Radiol.* 2001, 36(7):368-377.

[15] Henry-Feugeas MC, Idy-Peretti I, Baledent O, Poncelet-Didon A, Zannoli G, Bittoun J, Schouman-Claeys E: Origin of subarachnoid cerebrospinal fluid pulsations: a phase-contrast MR analysis. *Magn. Reson. Imaging* 2000, 18(4):387-395.

[16] Saliou G, Paradot G, Gondry C, Bouzerar R, Lehmann P, Meyers ME, Gars DL, Deramond H, Baledent O: A phase-contrast MRI study of acute and chronic hydrodynamic alterations after hydrocephalus induced by subarachnoid hemorrhage. *J Neuroimaging* 2012, 22(4):343-350.

[17] Germanwala AV, Huang J, Tamargo RJ: Hydrocephalus after aneurysmal subarachnoid hemorrhage. *Neurosurg. Clin. N. Am.* 2010, 21(2):263-270.

[18] Komotar RJ, Olivi A, Rigamonti D, Tamargo RJ: Microsurgical fenestration of the lamina terminalis reduces the incidence of shunt-dependent hydrocephalus after aneurysmal subarachnoid hemorrhage. *Neurosurgery* 2002, 51(6):1403-1412; discussion 1412-1403.

[19] Marlin AE, Wald A, Hochwald GM, Malhan C: Kaolin-induced hydrocephalus impairs CSF secretion by the choroid plexus. *Neurology* 1978, 28(9 Pt 1):945-949.

[20] Wald A, Hochwald GM, Malhan C: The effects of ventricular fluid osmolality on bulk flow of nascent fluid into the cerebral ventricles of cats. *Experimental brain research Experimentelle Hirnforschung Experimentation cerebrale* 1976, 25(2):157-167.

[21] Kanat A, Turkmenoglu O, Aydin MD, Yolas C, Aydin N, Gursan N, Tumkaya L, Demir R: Toward changing of the pathophysiologic basis of acute hydrocephalus after subarachnoid hemorrhage: a preliminary experimental study. *World neurosurgery* 2013, 80(3-4):390-395.

[22] Li J, McAllister JP, 2nd, Shen Y, Wagshul ME, Miller JM, Egnor MR, Johnston MG, Haacke EM, Walker ML: Communicating hydrocephalus in adult rats with kaolin obstruction of the basal cisterns or the cortical subarachnoid space. *Experimental neurology* 2008, 211(2):351-361.

[23] van Gijn J, Hijdra A, Wijdicks EF, Vermeulen M, van Crevel H: Acute hydrocephalus after aneurysmal subarachnoid hemorrhage. *Journal of neurosurgery* 1985, 63(3):355-362.

[24] Srinivasan VM, O'Neill BR, Jho D, Whiting DM, Oh MY: The history of external ventricular drainage. *Journal of neurosurgery* 2014, 120(1):228-236.

[25] Paine JT, Batjer HH, Samson D: Intraoperative ventricular puncture. *Neurosurgery* 1988, 22(6 Pt 1):1107-1109.

[26] Stangl AP, Meyer B, Zentner J, Schramm J: Continuous external CSF drainage--a perpetual problem in neurosurgery. *Surg. Neurol.* 1998, 50(1):77-82.

[27] Sussman ES, Kellner CP, Nelson E, McDowell MM, Bruce SS, Bruce RA, Zhuang Z, Connolly ES, Jr.: Hemorrhagic complications of ventriculostomy: incidence and predictors in patients with intracerebral hemorrhage. *Journal of neurosurgery* 2014, 120(4):931-936.

[28] Khanna RK, Rosenblum ML, Rock JP, Malik GM: Prolonged external ventricular drainage with percutaneous long-tunnel ventriculostomies. *Journal of neurosurgery* 1995, 83(5):791-794.

[29] Paramore CG, Turner DA: Relative risks of ventriculostomy infection and morbidity. *Acta Neurochir (Wien)* 1994, 127(1-2):79-84.

[30] Kakarla UK, Kim LJ, Chang SW, Theodore N, Spetzler RF: Safety and accuracy of bedside external ventricular drain placement. *Neurosurgery* 2008, 63(1 Suppl 1):ONS162-166; discussion ONS166-167.

[31] Ormond DR, Dressler A, Kim S, Ronecker J, Murali R: Lumbar drains may reduce the need for permanent CSF diversion in spontaneous subarachnoid hemorrhage. *Br. J. Neurosurg* 2013, 27(2):171-174.

[32] Al-Tamimi YZ, Bhargava D, Feltbower RG, Hall G, Goddard AJ, Quinn AC, Ross SA: Lumbar drainage of cerebrospinal fluid after aneurysmal subarachnoid hemorrhage: a prospective, randomized, controlled trial (LUMAS). *Stroke; a journal of cerebral circulation* 2012, 43(3):677-682.

[33] Grady RE, Horlocker TT, Brown RD, Maxson PM, Schroeder DR: Neurologic complications after placement of cerebrospinal fluid drainage catheters and needles in anesthetized patients: implications for regional anesthesia. Mayo Perioperative Outcomes Group. *Anesth Analg.* 1999, 88(2):388-392.

[34] Roland PS, Marple BF, Meyerhoff WL, Mickey B: Complications of lumbar spinal fluid drainage. *Otolaryngol Head Neck Surg.* 1992, 107(4):564-569.

[35] Hoekema D, Schmidt RH, Ross I: Lumbar drainage for subarachnoid hemorrhage: technical considerations and safety analysis. *Neurocritical care* 2007, 7(1):3-9.

[36] Houle PJ, Vender JR, Fountas K, McDonnell DE, Fick JR, Robinson JS: Pump-regulated lumbar subarachnoid drainage. *Neurosurgery* 2000, 46(4):929-932.

[37] Pleasure SJ, Abosch A, Friedman J, Ko NU, Barbaro N, Dillon W, Fishman RA, Poncelet AN: Spontaneous intracranial hypotension resulting in stupor caused by diencephalic compression. *Neurology* 1998, 50(6):1854-1857.

[38] Yasargil MG, Yonekawa Y, Zumstein B, Stahl HJ: Hydrocephalus following spontaneous subarachnoid hemorrhage. Clinical features and treatment. *Journal of neurosurgery* 1973, 39(4):474-479.

[39] Komotar RJ, Hahn DK, Kim GH, Starke RM, Garrett MC, Merkow MB, Otten ML, Sciacca RR, Connolly ES, Jr.: Efficacy of lamina terminalis fenestration in reducing shunt-dependent hydrocephalus following aneurysmal subarachnoid hemorrhage: a systematic review. Clinical article. *Journal of neurosurgery* 2009, 111(1):147-154.

[40] Obaid S, Weil AG, Rahme R, Bojanowski MW: Endoscopic Third Ventriculostomy for Obstructive Hydrocephalus due to Intraventricular Hemorrhage. *Journal of neurological surgery Part A, Central European neurosurgery* 2014.

[41] Fukuhara T, Shimizu T, Namba Y: Limited efficacy of endoscopic third ventriculostomy for hydrocephalus following aneurysmal subarachnoid hemorrhage. *Neurol. Med. Chir. (Tokyo)* 2009, 49(10):449-455.

[42] Klopfenstein JD, Kim LJ, Feiz-Erfan I, Hott JS, Goslar P, Zabramski JM, Spetzler RF: Comparison of rapid and gradual weaning from external ventricular drainage in patients with aneurysmal subarachnoid hemorrhage: a prospective randomized trial. *Journal of neurosurgery* 2004, 100(2):225-229.

[43] Olson DM, Zomorodi M, Britz GW, Zomorodi AR, Amato A, Graffagnino C: Continuous cerebral spinal fluid drainage associated with complications in patients admitted with subarachnoid hemorrhage. *Journal of neurosurgery* 2013, 119(4):974-980.

[44] Lee CK, Tay LL, Ng WH, Ng I, Ang BT: Optimization of ventricular catheter placement via posterior approaches: a virtual reality simulation study. *Surg. Neurol.* 2008, 70(3):274-277; discussion 277-278.

[45] Rammos S, Klopfenstein J, Augspurger L, Wang H, Wagenbach A, Poston J, Lanzino G: Conversion of external ventricular drains to ventriculoperitoneal shunts after aneurysmal subarachnoid hemorrhage: effects of site and protein/red blood cell counts on shunt infection and malfunction. *Journal of neurosurgery* 2008, 109(6):1001-1004.

[46] Sheth SA, McGirt M, Woodworth G, Wang P, Rigamonti D: Ultrasound guidance for distal insertion of ventriculo-atrial shunt catheters: technical note. *Neurological research* 2009, 31(3):280-282.

[47] Megison DP, Benzel EC: Ventriculo-pleural shunting for adult hydrocephalus. *Br. J. Neurosurg.* 1988, 2(4):503-505.

[48] Girotti ME, Singh RR, Rodgers BM: The ventriculo-gallbladder shunt in the treatment of refractory hydrocephalus: a review of the current literature. *The American surgeon* 2009, 75(8):734-737.

[49] Kang S: Efficacy of lumbo-peritoneal versus ventriculo-peritoneal shunting for management of chronic hydrocephalus following aneurysmal subarachnoid hemorrhage. *Acta Neurochir (Wien)* 2000, 142(1):45-49.

[50] Aoki N: Lumboperitoneal shunt: clinical applications, complications, and comparison with ventriculoperitoneal shunt. *Neurosurgery* 1990, 26(6):998-1003; discussion 1003-1004.

In: Subarachnoid Hemorrhage
Editor: Linda R. Gray
ISBN: 978-1-63463-492-2

Chapter 3

Subarachnoid Hemorrhage: Epidemiology, Management and New Approaches to Measure Outcome

Thomas Kapapa[1,•] and Ralph König[1]
[1]Department of Neurosurgery, University of Ulm, Ulm, Germany

Abstract

The spontaneous subarachnoid hemorrhage went through different changes and developments since one of its first description by Hippocrates of Cos. The last developments in management and treatment are represented by the introduction of early intervention in aneurysms within the first 72 hours after bleeding and the introduction of endovascular coiling and stenting techniques in the 90ies. However, challenges like permanent post haemorrhage hydrocephalus, the delayed cerebral ischemia with the angiographic phenomenon of vasospasms, and cognitive deficits with impaired health-related quality of life are still present. The last and recent decade provided a sophisticated debate about the preferable treatment options within surgical and endovascular manoeuvres, especially in incidental aneurysms. When it seemed that the pendulum went to the side of endovascular treatment it recently seems to

• Tel.: +49 731 500 55001, Fax: +49 731 500 55002, E-mail: Thomas.Kapapa@uniklinik-ulm.de.

come back to surgical options. New technical achievements like neuronaviagtion and hybrid surgical theatres found the way into the field and contributed. Knowledge about the molecular and biochemical background of vasospasms and the clinical overall picture as delayed cerebral ischemia increased. This resulted in new treatment points like the continuously intra atrial given calcium channel blockers. Nevertheless, major aim is to improve the outcome for the patient with a new view including his neurocognitive and his mental conditions and to reduce his physical and psychological long term impairments.

Introduction

Rather than being an isolated, fateful occurrence, spontaneous subarachnoid hemorrhage is an epidemiologically relevant condition with an incidence of 5%-10% amongst all cases of stroke [1]. The number of those affected in Germany is not known, but in the USA is estimated at 25,000 to 32,000 [2, 3]. Despite advances in endovascular therapy and diagnostic techniques, as well as in perioperative care, the current mortality rates remain very poor, at up to 45% [4-7]. Morbidity is high, reaching 80% [2, 8-13]. Scientific research to date has not delivered any convincing results as regards an improvement in this unsatisfactory situation. Since the switch to rapid treatment for subarachnoid hemorrhage in the 1990s and introduction of endovascular treatment, there have been few further therapeutic improvements with a view to optimising the mortality and morbidity rates [14-16]. The main cause for death and morbidity after subarachnoid hemorrhage at present is cerebral vasospasm [17].

Incidence of Spontaneous Aneurysmal Subarachnoid Hemorrhage

Regional differences are evident in the incidence of spontaneous aneurysmal subarachnoid hemorrhage, with figures reported at 2 to 32 per 100,000 inhabitants. This more than ten-fold difference is noticeable in particular between China and Japan [18, 19]. In Europe, rates of 10 to 23 per 100,000 inhabitants have been reported [7, 18]. No recent figures are available for the most of European countries.

Incidence increases with age. The condition mainly occurs between the ages of 40 and 60 year; women aged 40 to 50 years are more likely to be affected. The rate levels out again between the ages of 50 and 60. In total, women are affected 1.2 to 1.6 times more than men [8, 18, 20, 21]. The rate tends to increase in individuals over 65 years of age [4-6].

Risk Factors for Spontaneous Subarachnoid Hemorrhage

Numerous risk factors have been identified for subarachnoid hemorrhage. Multivariate analysis revealed smoking, excessive alcohol consumption and hypertension as independent risk factors [22-29]. However, current publications present a new score for rating the risk of the rupture risk of an intact aneurysm. 1.4% and 3.4% was determined for the mean one-year and five-year risk for ruptured aneurysm, respectively. Predictors for rupture were age, existing hypertension, a history of Subarachnoid Hemorrhage, the size of the aneurysm, the localisation of the aneurysm, and the geographic area in which the subjects lived. In North America and Europe (with the exception of Finland), the absolute five-year risk for a ruptured cerebral aneurysm ranged from 0.25% for those under 70 years of age with no vascular risk factors and a small internal carotid artery aneurysm (< 7 mm), to more than 15% for patients over 70 years with hypertension, a history of subarachnoid hemorrhage as well as a very large aneurysm (> 20 mm) in the posterior circulation. Compared to subjects in North America and in European nations (excepting Finland), the rupture risk of aneurysms was 3.6 times higher in the Finnish and 2.8 times higher in the Japanese population [30].

Earlier studies showed additionally sympathomimetic drugs, cocaine and phenylpropanolamine as further risk factors [31-34]. In a number of studies, no significant correlation could be found between meteorological events and subarachnoid hemorrhage. At most, weak correlations could be found between a change in atmospheric pressure ranges, atmospheric pressures, and the daily incidence of subarachnoid hemorrhage [35-40].

Of the genetic risks factors, autosomal dominant congenital polycystic kidney disease and Ehlers-Danlos syndrome type IV are to mention [41-51]. Here, the risk of aneurysm rupture was rated as approx. 8% (relative risk of about 4.2%) [52, 53]. The risk of experiencing aneurysmal subarachnoid hemorrhage is higher if at least one family members have already suffered such an event [53]. The occurrence of asymptomatic aneurysms in a study using magnetic resonance imaging was approx. 7%. This figure increased to 10.5% in individuals with a relative who had suffered subarachnoid hemorrhage [54]. Yet, no specific gene could be identified, however, nor could any single nucleotide polymorphism be found to correlate with the spontaneous subarachnoid hemorrhage [55].

It has been ascertained that the risk of a new aneurysm developing subsequent to subarachnoid hemorrhage is 1% to 2% per year. Patients with multiple aneurysms appear to have a higher risk of developing new aneurysms [49, 51, 56-62].

Manifestation of Spontaneous Subarachnoid Hemorrhage

The majority of patients (80%) describe the hemorrhagic event as excruciating headaches of indescribable magnitude. A further 20% describe preceding headaches [63-65]. Most intracranial aneurysms remain asymptomatic until they rupture. This can happen at any time, though mostly in conjunction with physical exertion [66, 67]. Headache is not the only symptom: it can be accompanied by nausea and vomiting (77%), meningism (35%), impaired consciousness as far as coma (53%) and focal neurological deficits (cranial nerve dysfunction) [8]. Seizures (focal or generalised) occur in up to 20% of subarachnoid hemorrhages as a direct result of the bleeding, especially within the first 24 hours [68]. The occurrence of a seizure is a poor prognostic sign in terms of health-related quality of life [69].

Diagnostics after Subarachnoid Hemorrhage

If acute subarachnoid hemorrhage is suspected, computed cranial tomography is the imaging method of choice. Computed tomographic angiography is fast, readily available, and – with the exception of applying the contrast agent – non-invasive. Contemporary methods of computed tomography angiography reveal a sensitivity to larger aneurysms ($\geq$ 5 mm) which is similar to that of selective catheter angiography, up to 100%. Specificity is reported as also up to 100% [50, 70-75]. Due to resorption and redistribution processes, however, its sensitivity drops significantly within the initial days following haemorrhage: 98%-100% immediately after the event, up to 93% within the first 24 hours, 85% within the first 5 days, and less than 30% after 2 weeks, respectively [76, 77]. Magnetic resonance imaging is exceptionally valuable in the detection of subacute subarachnoid hemorrhage, but in the acute phase is not usually the imaging method of choice due to the time and logistical efforts involved [78]. Sensitivity is 85%-100% in an aneurysm measuring 5 mm, but drops when the aneurysm measures less than 5 mm [79-82]. However, the sensitivity and specificity of computed tomography angiography depend on the localisation and size of the aneurysm, experience of the examiner, data acquisition and software for data presentation. Given a characteristic history but no imaging evidence of bleeding, lumbar puncture is still regarded as obligatory for ruling out subarachnoid hemorrhage [77, 83].

To identify the cause for the haemorrhage, selective panangiography remains the criterion standard. Continual technical advancements in sectional imaging, however, have now made CT angiography, in particular, the imaging technique of choice. Its sensitivity, or specificity respectively, is very high, though it lessens as the size of the aneurysm grows [84].

Preoperative Assessment Treatment for Spontaneous Subarachnoid Hemorrhage

Once the vital parameters have stabilised, rapid transfer to the nearest and most suitable hospital (with neurosurgical support) is crucial to survival. Numerous classification systems are in place for assessing the clinical picture. Examples are the Hunt & Hess Scale, Fisher Score, Glasgow Coma Score and the World Federation of Neurological Surgeons Score (WFNS) [85-88]. There are shortcomings in these assessments, since they are mostly performed retrospectively, i.e. after intubation. The difference in the intraindividual and interindividual assessment can also lead to errors [89, 90].

Secondary Bleeding after Subarachnoid Hemorrhage

A fast and decided therapeutic strategy is required if secondary bleeding is to be avoided [91-96]. The sooner the source of the bleeding is localised and sealed, the lower the risk of secondary hemorrhage (Table 1) [14, 15, 97-101]. If this is not possible, the systolic blood pressure should be maintained at below 150 mm Hg [102, 103]. Bed rest is essential, though alone it is not a guarantee against the onset of secondary bleeding [93].

Table 1. Frequency of secondary hemorrhage in untreated aneurysms [15]

Days after hemorrhage	Frequency of secondary hemorrhage
0 – 3	5.7%
4 – 6	9.4%
7 – 10	12.7%
11 - 14	13.9%
15 - 32	21.5%

Endovascular and Microsurgical Treatment of Aneurysmal Subarachnoid Hemorrhage

Due to the high rate of secondary bleeding from ruptured cerebral aneurysms in the first few days after the hemorrhage has occurred, early treatment of the cerebral aneurysms has – with few exceptions – become firmly established [14, 15, 95, 104, 105]. As far as the 1990s, microsurgery for cerebral aneurysms was regarded as the treatment of choice. The publication of reports by Guglielmi on electrolytically detachable platinum coils for endovascular occlusion of aneurysms changed the face of aneurysm treatment dramatically [106-110]. Today, the ratio of endovascular to microsurgical treatments of ruptured aneurysms at most neurovascular centres is at least 60:40. The appropriate therapeutic concept for each individual aneurysm is generally determined on an interdisciplinary level, whereby various factors are important: institutional set-up, localisation and configuration of the aneurysm, and patient-relevant factors such as age or clinical condition, to name but a few.

In 1991, Guglielmi et al. presented a method with which to occlude intracranial aneurysms endovascularly using electrolytically detachable platinum coils [106, 107]. In doing so, the lumen of the aneurysm is compacted by the coil and thus occluded following thrombosis. The risk from the endovascular method is estimated at between 2.4% (perforation) and 8.5% (procedural ischaemias) [111, 112]. The combination of morbidity and mortality after endovascular treatment is up to 25.4% (mortality after surgical clipping is up to 30.6%) [16]. Procedural mortality is reported as up to 2%, and the incidence of physical disabilities up to 7.4% for the first 30 days [16, 113, 114]. The reperfusion rate after endovascular occlusion of an aneurysm is reported at between 0% and 50% [60, 115-124]. Often, the resulting secondary bleeding is lethal [122]. Secondary hemorrhaging following endovascular occlusion of an aneurysm is reported at a rate of approx. 2.9% [16, 113]. The probability of secondary bleeding is highest in the first 12 months [125].

Meta-analysis of the published data demonstrates that complete occlusion of an aneurysm is very difficult to achieve. For example, only 55% of treated aneurysms are completely occluded and 88% are occluded by more than 90% [111, 126].

Some aneurysms are difficult to treat endovascularly due to anatomy (e.g. medial cerebral artery) [127-130]. In such cases, surgery is estimated more successful than the endovascular technique [131-133]. Conversely, aneurysms in the posterior circle of Willis and cavernous sinus are more difficult to manage surgically, and so endovascular therapy delivers better results [52, 134-137]. Comorbidities and factors related to the initial hemorrhage are further criteria which indicate surgical or interventional treatment of an aneurysm. Intraparenchymal bleeding with mass impact, for example, is an indication for surgery. If the neurological status is poor or there is evidence of intracranial swelling, surgery should not be undertaken due to the retraction of parts of the brain [138, 139].

Complete surgical occlusion of an aneurysm is achieved in about 92% of cases. In such aneurysms, a reperfusion rate of 0.5% with no secondary hemorrhage is reported. In incompletely occluded aneurysms, a reperfusion rate of about 3% to 4% per year is reported, whereby the rate of secondary bleeding is approximately 1.5%. In all surgically occluded aneurysms – irrespective of residual perfusion – the risk of secondary hemorrhage is 0.26% [60, 140]. The rate of post-interventional, secondary hemorrhage, when comparing the surgical and endovascular method, is 0.9% with clipping and 2.9% with coiling [16, 113].

When comparing the treatment outcomes of surgical and endovascular approaches, the initial neurological status of the patient proves important [12, 141]. From an annual perspective, there is hardly any difference in the mortality rate between endovascular (8.1%) and surgical (10.1%) management [16, 113]. The morbidity rates of 21.6% from the surgical and 15.6% from the endovascular approach suggest that the endovascular technique is advantageous. The absolute risk in this case is 30.9% (clipping) versus 23.5% (coiling), with a significance of p=0.0001. The rate of secondary hemorrhage was 2.9% from endovascular and 0.9% from surgical treatment [16, 113]. The question whether such an advantage is maintained over several years is being investigated.

Cerebral Vasospasm after Spontaneous Subarachnoid Hemorrhage

Aside from the severity of the initial hemorrhage, cerebral vasospasm plays a decisive role in the prognosis of the spontaneous subarachnoid hemorrhage. It occurs in 30% to 70%, primarily in young and in female patients, between the third and fifth day post hemorrhage, in particular. There are suggestions that vasospasm and late-onset infarcts occur less often after endovascular treatment of an aneurysm [142]. At present, as many as 20% of patients die from the ischaemic complications resulting from cerebral vasospasm, despite intensive medicine [143, 144]. It is very important that vasospasms will be detected, especially in the first 14 days following the hemorrhagic event. Aside from routine clinical follow-up examinations in the alert patient, Doppler ultrasound, tissue oxygen partial pressure measurement and MR or CT perfusion imaging scans are of great importance [144, 145]. Drug based vasospasm prophylaxis with nimodipine, preferably oral or otherwise intravenous, is a treatment commensurate with the relevant guidelines [77]. In recent years, interventional treatment methods are increasingly being used as rescue therapies for refractory cerebral vasospasm [146, 147].

A cerebral vasospasm is a narrowing of the intracranial arteries. Clinically there is a deterioration in the patient's condition, and radiologically a reduction in cerebral perfusion. Cerebral vasospasm occurs at a rate of 30% - 70% between days 3 to 5 post subarachnoid hemorrhage, and peaks after 5 to 14 days [148, 149]. Up to 20% of patients with cerebral vasospasm are lost to ischaemic complications despite receiving therapy [150, 151]. Meanwhile, up to 50% of patients suffering subarachnoid hemorrhage die from cerebral vasospasm [95]. Aside from focal neurological deficits which cannot be explained by impaired circulation of the cerebrospinal fluid or secondary bleeding, an increase in mean arterial pressure (signifying cerebral autoregulation in the presence of perfusion deficits) is an indication of vasospasm.

Transcranial Doppler is not free of controversy, however, since the results depend on the examiner [152-154]. Incorrect values may be captured during hypertensive therapy for vasospasm [155-158]. The criterion standard for diagnosis of cerebral vasospasm is digital subtraction angiography [159, 160].

Effective prophylaxis and therapy for cerebral vasospasm begin with eliminating the source of the bleeding; hemodynamic methods permit early and aggressive treatment of the cerebral vasospasm [161]. The goal of the prophylactic and therapeutic measures in the case of cerebral vasospasm is to reduce the risk of cerebral ischaemia by controlling intracranial pressure, decreasing the cerebral oxygen consumption and improving cerebral blood flow. The prophylactic benefit of hypervolaemia as opposed to normovolaemia is still debated.

Calcium channel blockers predominate in the prophylaxis and treatment of cerebral vasospasm. They are claimed to reduce morbidity and improve the functional treatment outcome. No evidence of a physical reduction in vasospasm has been found. Thus, improved perfusion is described as advantageous [162, 163]. Unlike nimodipine, intravenous nicardipine revealed a 30% reduction in vasospasm but no improvement in the treatment outcome [164].

The introduction of nicardipine pellets into the basal cisterns has likewise demonstrated positive effects [165]. The number needed to treat, according to current literature, remains at 19 [166, 167].

Other methods, such as medicinal augmentation of fibrinolysis, acetylsalicylic acid, enoxaparin, tirilazad, nitroglycerin, endothelin-1a antagonists, statins and moderate shaking of the head to dissolve the blood clot, have been found in part to reduce mortality and/or morbidity. They have not yet found their way into the armamentarium of intensive medicine [168-180]. Endovascular therapy for vasospasm, using angioplasty, has resulted in decreased mortality following vasospasm [181]. The strategic objective is to increase cerebral blood flow distal to the stenosis. Balloon angioplasty for mechanical dilatation of spastic intracranial arteries, using a microcatheter, was first reported in 1984.

Dilatation is most effective in large proximal vessels with thick, muscular walls. It is less effective and safe, however, in distal perforator vessels behind the secondary segmental arteries [182-185]. Papaverine or nimodipine should be used in these blood vessels [186-190]. Risks from brain stem depression, hypotension, aggravation of vasospasm, seizures, respiratory disorders, hemipareses or increased intracranial pressure are rare during a slow infusion [188, 191]. Balloon angioplasty and infusion of vasodilators can take place in one session. A superior effect in terms of the treatment outcome has not been identified [192, 193].

The selection of suitable patients and the appropriate timing for endovascular treatment of vasospasm is currently being studied. Angioplasty will not deliver a positive effect in every patient. Studies are ongoing in which suitable patients are being selected on the basis of diagnostic imaging, using perfusion deficit measurements in computed tomography and magnetic resonance imaging [194-197].

Impaired CSF Circulation and Hydrocephalus after Spontaneous Subarachnoid Hemorrhage

Acute hydrocephalus occurs in up to 80% of all cases of spontaneous subarachnoid hemorrhage. Treatment is administered on the basis of the neuroradiological picture by inserting a ventricular or lumbar drain. Up to 30% of patients require permanent CSF drainage; predictors here, aside from the volume and distribution of the blood, are the duration of external CSF drainage, the occurrence of meningitis over the course of treatment, and the anatomic position of the aneurysm. Hence, patients with aneurysms in the vertebral artery appear to require permanent CSF drainage much more often than those with aneurysms in the medial cerebral artery [198]. CSF drainage in the acute phase of a subarachnoid hemorrhage has a protective effect with respect to cerebral vasospasm [199, 200].

Seizures after Spontaneous Subarachnoid Hemorrhage

Seizures after subarachnoid hemorrhage are a negative predictor for health-related quality of life [69]. The frequency of cerebral seizures is reported at between 6% and 18% [201-203]. Most often, they occur prior to the arrival of medical assistance. In the hospital, seizures are reported at a rate of about 7% [204]. Risk factors for seizures are aneurysms in the medial cerebral artery, intraparenchymal haematomas, infarctions and hypertension [205-210]. The benefit of prophylactic anticonvulsive therapy is not known [211-213].

Hemicraniectomy as a Treatment for Refractory Intracranial Hypertension after Spontaneous Subarachnoid Hemorrhage

The benefit of decompressive craniectomy to spontaneous subarachnoid hemorrhage is more highly disputed than the benefit offered to severe cerebral ischaemias or traumatic brain injuries [214-216]. Decompressive hemicraniectomy appears to result in decreased morbidity in the case of subarachnoid hemorrhage with intraparenchymal bleeding, and mainly in reduced mortality in the case of refractory cerebral hypertension [217-219].

Treatment Outcome after Spontaneous Subarachnoid Hemorrhage

A differentiated approach must be taken when assessing the treatment outcome. The factors that influence the treatment outcome can be divided into three categories:

A) Patient-related factors:
    Severity of bleeding, clinical condition on admission, age, sex, time until treatment, comorbities, risk factors [4]
B) Aneurysm and hemorrhage-related factors, clinical course:
    Size of the aneurysm, localisation, morphology, vasospasm, hydrocephalus, secondary hemorrhage etc. [220]
C) Institutional factors:
    First treating hospital, diagnostic methods, clinical experience with the disease, endovascular treatment options [4, 127, 134, 220, 221]

The assessment of the therapeutic outcome in itself must satisfy criteria which account for the varying degrees of hemorrhage severity, the treatment options and care directives, as well as patient-associated circumstances before, during and after treatment. This means that a contemporary assessment of the treatment outcome must represent a sum of the judgements made by the doctors, paramedics, and the patients themselves. Patients are not very well served if the doctor offers an assessment to the effect of "good or very good functional treatment outcome after severe subarachnoid hemorrhage", whereby, for instance, the patient has given up his executive job due to headaches and cognitive deficits, and there have been negative effects on the family.

The path of knowledge described here is the result of an historical process that was focused primarily on patients surviving a spontaneous subarachnoid hemorrhage. This is recognised from the fact that in older publications, aspects such as quality of life or cognition are seldom mentioned [141]. Today, such aspects are more or less a prerequisite.

Historical Criteria for Assessing Treatment Outcome

Survival

The greatest influence on the rate of survivors has been achieved by means of innovative changes in the management and introduction of technology and techniques (Figure 1). This applies in particular to the introduction of microsurgery, computed tomography in the diagnostic field, and a rapid surgical response (within 72 hours after onset of the hemorrhage), as well as the possibility of endovascular treatment and prophylaxis with nimodipine [14, 15, 101, 106, 107, 161, 222-225]. Recent studies have demonstrated that mortality after one month is about 33%. Compared with the results reported in the 1960s (death of approx. 33% of patients before reaching the hospital, death in 27% during treatment, or residual, severe physical impairments following treatment [42, 226]), there has been a clear improvement in the survival rate.

Institutional Factors

It has been suggested that there is a correlation between the treatment outcome and experience of the hospital in treating the condition [4, 181, 221, 227].

Experience with endovascular diagnostic and therapeutic methods plays an important role [4]. Hospitals with neurovascular and neuroradiological expertise that treat more than 35 cases per year have a much lower rate of mortality [4, 181].

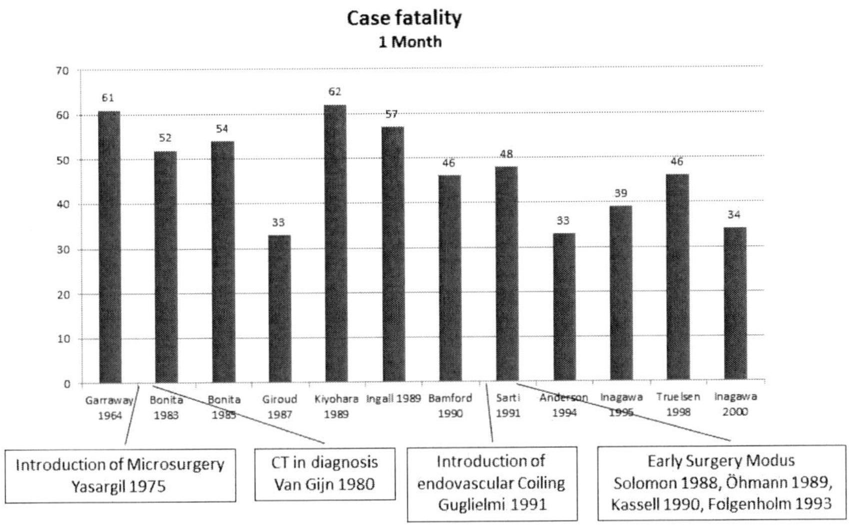

Figure 1. Presentation of the rate of fatal treatment procedures over time with influential innovations [6, 14, 15, 46, 101, 106, 107, 161, 222-225, 272-281].

Glasgow Outcome Scale

The Glasgow Outcome Scale, or modified Rankin Scale, is most commonly used as a means of assessing the treatment outcome [228-230]. Not only is the rate of those surviving spontaneous subarachnoid hemorrhage increasing, but also the number of patients with a good treatment outcome (Figure 2) [231].

This is likewise a reflection of the impact of technological advancements. Over the further course, the treatment outcome following spontaneous subarachnoid hemorrhage is often categorised in the literature and by clinicians in simple terms such as "good", "moderate" or "poor" for the purposes of rapid grading. Such judgements were made on the basis of the prevailing functional, neurological deficits, however, leaving little room for psychological, cognitive and social components. The quality of life of many patients, despite their physical well-being, may still be impaired (Figure 3). It is not unusual to find that neuropsychological and cognitive deficits are causing such impairments (Figure 4) [232, 233].

A spontaneous subarachnoid hemorrhage is a life-threatening condition and therefore can have a decisive influence on subsequent, health-related quality of life.

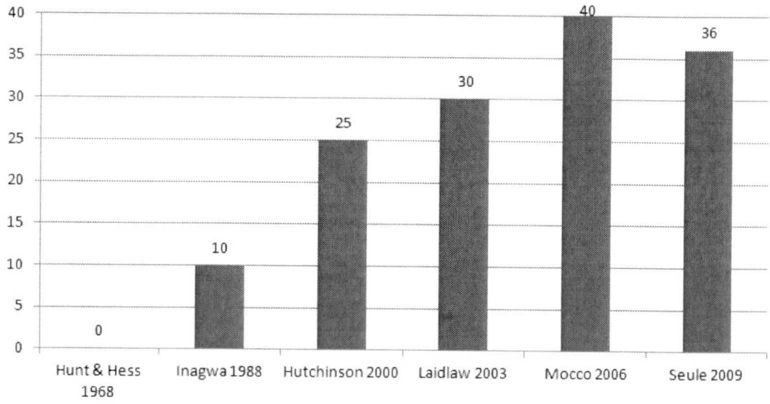

Figure 2. Proportion (%) of patients with good outcome according to the Glasgow Outcome Scale (GOS 4-5) [231].

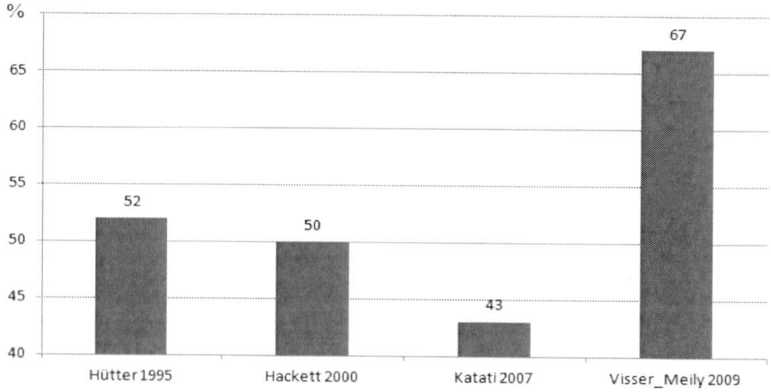

Figure 3. Proportion (%) of patients with impaired quality of life [241, 282-284].

Contemporary Criteria for Assessing Treatment Outcome

Quality of Life

Quality of life is a general buzzword that encompasses all the factors leading to happiness and satisfaction. The term is an attempt to describe the individual degree of personal satisfaction.

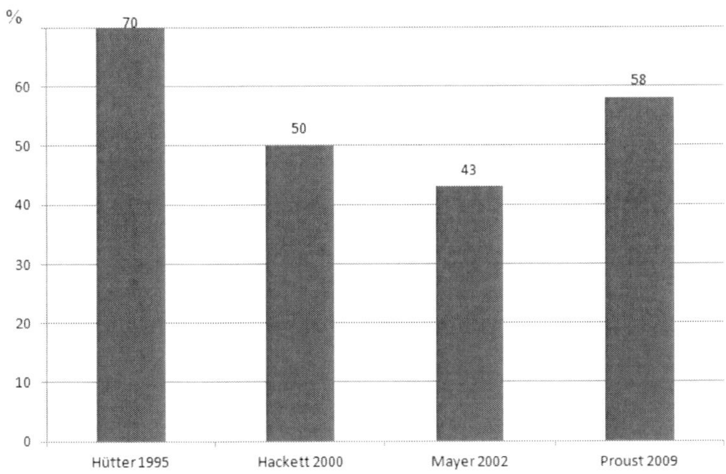

Figure 4. Proportion (%) of patients with cognitive dysfunctions and impaired quality of life [241, 248, 282, 285].

In medicine, the term "health-related quality of life" covers a number of criteria that aim to approximate a definition. Objectives, values and principles are encompassed by these criteria, e.g. the certainty and length of a lifetime and a specific standard of health, the freedom to seize opportunities, or personal and social recognition. Yet health-related quality of life is also influenced by other determinants, such as the existence of economic conditions for achieving the ideals placed upon a society or goals it has set for itself.

In the pursuit of holistic medicine, clinical endpoints are to be understood in the context of subjective satisfaction, psychosocial interaction and forward-looking behaviour. When discharging the patient, the clinical outcome should not merely extend as far as the door of the hospital. It should, rather, be judged in conjunction with the patient's customary family life, social ties and social integration, as well as the physical and mental capacity to achieve one's goals. Clinical parameters alone are not enough.

In the past, the clinical outcome, in the form of the physical "outcome", was deemed sufficient. It was described in terms of the clinical status on discharge. A disease can change a person's life over quite a long period, however. The treatment outcome is therefore an integrated part of the individual's situation. To gain insights into such a situation, health-related quality of life is a useful guide. It is a reflection of the disease, the result of treatment and the circumstances of life. It places the "patient" above the "disease", and also establishes a connection between the two. This provides the opportunity to compare rational health indications, objective clinical ratings and progress against the subjective views and treatment outcomes of the patient.

Health-related quality of life from patient-oriented medical care should serve as the criterion for the treatment outcome. Medical care that on the basis of its major technological advances must define new goals, tasks and limits [234].

Given the subjective description of the treatment outcome from the perspective of the patient, health-related quality of life supplements the "organic" treatment outcome. Related to a specific disease, it describes a therapeutic endpoint, for instance, based on one value.

Cognition

As far as cognitive function following spontaneous subarachnoid hemorrhage is concerned, the pivotal preliminary research was conducted in the 1990s by the study team of Hutter and Gilsbach [235-241]. There is a general consensus that cognitive deficits persist after spontaneous subarachnoid hemorrhage, outliving any improvements in residual physical deficits and ultimately leading to a permanent reduction in health-related quality of life [237, 241-245]. Very often they affect verbal memory, motor skills, executive (problem-solving) functions, visuo-spatial functions and visual memory, and take longest to recover [240, 246-250]. A good physical treatment outcome does not preclude cognitive deficits [237, 239, 241, 244, 251-253]. Cerebral bleeding causes marked changes in cognitive function [254]. Humans can to some extent compensate for such changes, though this depends on a variety of factors, including the severity and localisation of the bleeding, age and premorbid functioning. Some studies have examined the outcomes of treatment and, in particular, health-related quality of life following spontaneous subarachnoid hemorrhage [11, 69, 237, 241, 255-257]. Some examined the potentials of cognitive performance – structures and processes of attention, thought, emotion, memory, learning, motivation and perception.

The relevant data were obtained mainly from patients having undergone surgery and those prior to standardised endovascular therapy. It was postulated that endovascular therapy is the less aggressive option since it involves neither procedures that penetrate the skull nor temporary vascular occlusion, suggesting that post-interventional quality of life and cognition would be improved as a result [258-261]. This could not be entirely substantiated, however.

Neuropsychological deficits (irritability, isolation, aggression, disorientation, depression, lack of concentration, etc.) were documented in 42% - 65% of cases following subarachnoid hemorrhage. Such deficits can result in long-term morbidity and diminished social competence [241, 250]. Their incidence can cause the treatment outcome to be impaired, though this is seldom considered routinely.

A correlation between different aneurysmal localisations or "endovascular versus surgical therapy" could not be confirmed by more recent studies due to conflicting results. Vasospasm (with symptoms of headache) was found to have just as little impact [246, 262]. There was also no correlation between the scope of the cognitive impairments after spontaneous subarachnoid hemorrhage and radiological findings of focal cerebral lesions [263, 264]. Since no association could be found between focal lesions and localisation of the bleeding, it is presumed that the initial global increase in intracranial pressure causes diffuse damage [240, 262, 265, 266]. Nevertheless, the influence exerted by infarctions shows that patients with left-sided or bilateral medial/basal infarcts in particular experience difficulties with the verbal components of their memory [247, 267, 268]. However, the literature reveals that there is an inverse association between the duration of ventilation and psychomotor skills and memory [246]. The duration of mechanical ventilation reflects not only the impact of the hemorrhage, but more so the overall effect of the bleeding, the intraoperative and postoperative effects, as well as the methods of intensive care (prolonged ventilation, "coma healing") [269]. It must be noted, as a limitation, that some of these studies were conducted using computed tomography. Smaller lesions relevant when taken together and which can be identified by magnetic resonance imaging, were not detected. In summary, it is still postulated in the literature that the initial hemorrhage itself has the greatest influence on residual cognitive factors [244, 270]. This hypothesis is confirmed by the realisation that patients undergoing surgery for spontaneous subarachnoid hemorrhage have more severe cognitive impairments than patients having undergone surgery with incidental aneurysms [271].

Knowledge gained in the last decade has led to the development of cognitive rehabilitation concepts. This has resulted in the training of basic functions, though cognitive deficits persist. Studies performed 3, 6 and 12 months after spontaneous subarachnoid hemorrhage have demonstrated that verbal memory only improves from the second to the third test point. Executive functions, verbal intelligence and visual memory continually improved, whereas attention skills did not [246].

References

[1] Bederson, J. B., et al., Guidelines for the management of aneurysmal subarachnoid hemorrhage: a statement for healthcare professionals from a special writing group of the Stroke Council, American Heart Association. *Stroke,* 2009. 40(3): p. 994-1025.

[2] Shea, A. M., et al., Characteristics of nontraumatic subarachnoid hemorrhage in the United States in 2003. *Neurosurgery*, 2007. 61(6): p. 1131-7; discussion 1137-8.

[3] Diringer, M. N., Management of aneurysmal subarachnoid hemorrhage. *Crit. Care Med.,* 2009. 37(2): p. 432-40.

[4] Cross, D. T., 3rd, et al., Mortality rates after subarachnoid hemorrhage: variations according to hospital case volume in 18 states. *J. Neurosurg.,* 2003. 99(5): p. 810-7.

[5] Harmsen, P., A. Tsipogianni, and L. Wilhelmsen, Stroke incidence rates were unchanged, while fatality rates declined, during 1971-1987 in Goteborg, Sweden. *Stroke,* 1992. 23(10): p. 1410-5.

[6] Ingall, T. J., et al., Has there been a decline in subarachnoid hemorrhage mortality? *Stroke,* 1989. 20(6): p. 718-24.

[7] Stegmayr, B., M. Eriksson, and K. Asplund, Declining mortality from subarachnoid hemorrhage: changes in incidence and case fatality from 1985 through 2000. *Stroke,* 2004. 35(9): p. 2059-63.

[8] van Gijn, J. and G. J. Rinkel, Subarachnoid hemorrhage: diagnosis, causes and management. *Brain,* 2001. 124(Pt 2): p. 249-78.

[9] Hijdra, A., et al., Prediction of delayed cerebral ischemia, rebleeding, and outcome after aneurysmal subarachnoid hemorrhage. *Stroke*, 1988. 19(10): p. 1250-6.

[10] Hijdra, A., et al., Aneurysmal subarachnoid hemorrhage. Complications and outcome in a hospital population. *Stroke,* 1987. 18(6): p. 1061-7.

[11] Hop, J. W., et al., Changes in functional outcome and quality of life in patients and caregivers after aneurysmal subarachnoid hemorrhage. *J. Neurosurg.*, 2001. 95(6): p. 957-63.

[12] Broderick, J. P., et al., Initial and recurrent bleeding are the major causes of death following subarachnoid hemorrhage. *Stroke,* 1994. 25(7): p. 1342-7.

[13] Sundt, T. M., Jr., et al., Results and complications of surgical management of 809 intracranial aneurysms in 722 cases. Related and unrelated to grade of patient, type of aneurysm, and timing of surgery. *J. Neurosurg.*, 1982. 56(6): p. 753-65.

[14] Kassell, N. F., et al., The International Cooperative Study on the Timing of Aneurysm Surgery. Part 1: Overall management results. *J. Neurosurg.*, 1990. 73(1): p. 18-36.

[15] Kassell, N. F., et al., The International Cooperative Study on the Timing of Aneurysm Surgery. Part 2: Surgical results. *J. Neurosurg.*, 1990. 73(1): p. 37-47.

[16] Molyneux, A., et al., International Subarachnoid Aneurysm Trial (ISAT) of neurosurgical clipping versus endovascular coiling in 2143 patients with ruptured intracranial aneurysms: a randomised trial. *Lancet,* 2002. 360(9342): p. 1267-74.

[17] Harrod, C. G., B. R. Bendok, and H. H. Batjer, Prediction of cerebral vasospasm in patients presenting with aneurysmal subarachnoid hemorrhage: a review. *Neurosurgery,* 2005. 56(4): p. 633-54; discussion 633-54.

[18] Ingall, T., et al., A multinational comparison of subarachnoid hemorrhage epidemiology in the WHO MONICA stroke study. *Stroke,* 2000. 31(5): p. 1054-61.

[19] Inagawa, T., What are the actual incidence and mortality rates of subarachnoid hemorrhage? *Surg. Neurol.*, 1997. 47(1): p. 47-52; discussion 52-3.

[20] Eden, S. V., et al., Gender and ethnic differences in subarachnoid hemorrhage. *Neurology,* 2008. 71(10): p. 731-5.

[21] Rinkel, G. J., et al., Prevalence and risk of rupture of intracranial aneurysms: a systematic review. *Stroke,* 1998. 29(1): p. 251-6.

[22] Qureshi, A. I., et al., Cocaine use and hypertension are major risk factors for intracerebral hemorrhage in young African Americans. *Ethn. Dis.*, 2001. 11(2): p. 311-9.

[23] Qureshi, A. I., et al., Risk factors for subarachnoid hemorrhage. *Neurosurgery,* 2001. 49(3): p. 607-12; discussion 612-3.

[24] Taylor, C. L., et al., Cerebral arterial aneurysm formation and rupture in 20,767 elderly patients: hypertension and other risk factors. *J. Neurosurg.*, 1995. 83(5): p. 812-9.

[25] Kubota, M., A. Yamaura, and J. Ono, Prevalence of risk factors for aneurysmal subarachnoid hemorrhage: results of a Japanese multicentre case control study for stroke. *Br. J. Neurosurg.*, 2001. 15(6): p. 474-8.

[26] van der Schaaf, I. C., et al., Study design and outcome measures in studies on aneurysmal subarachnoid hemorrhage. *Stroke*, 2002. 33(8): p. 2043-6.

[27] Teunissen, L. L., et al., Risk factors for subarachnoid hemorrhage: a systematic review. *Stroke,* 1996. 27(3): p. 544-9.

[28] Knekt, P., et al., Risk factors for subarachnoid hemorrhage in a longitudinal population study. *J. Clin. Epidemiol.*, 1991. 44(9): p. 933-9.

[29] Juvela, S., et al., Cigarette smoking and alcohol consumption as risk factors for aneurysmal subarachnoid hemorrhage. *Stroke*, 1993. 24(5): p. 639-46.

[30] Greving, J. P., et al., Development of the PHASES score for prediction of risk of rupture of intracranial aneurysms: a pooled analysis of six prospective cohort studies. *Lancet Neurol.*, 2014. 13(1): p. 59-66.

[31] Moussouttas, M., Cannabis use and cerebrovascular disease. *Neurologist,* 2004. 10(1): p. 47-53.

[32] Nanda, A., et al., Intracranial aneurysms and cocaine abuse: analysis of prognostic indicators. *Neurosurgery,* 2000. 46(5): p. 1063-7; discussion 1067-9.

[33] Oyesiku, N. M., et al., Cocaine-induced aneurysmal rupture: an emergent negative factor in the natural history of intracranial aneurysms? *Neurosurgery*, 1993. 32(4): p. 518-25; discussion 525-6.

[34] Kernan, W. N., et al., Phenylpropanolamine and the risk of hemorrhagic stroke. *N. Engl. J. Med.,* 2000. 343(25): p. 1826-32.

[35] BTF Brain Trauma Foundation, A.A.o.N.S.A., Joint Section on Neurotrauma and Critical Care, Guidelines for the management of severe head injury. *J. Neurotrauma,* 2000. 14: p. 457-462.

[36] Inagawa, T., Seasonal variation in the incidence of aneurysmal subarachnoid hemorrhage in hospital- and community-based studies. *J. Neurosurg.*, 2002. 96(3): p. 497-509.

[37] Gallerani, M., et al., Circadian and circannual rhythmicity in the occurrence of subarachnoid hemorrhage. *Stroke,* 1996. 27(10): p. 1793-7.

[38] Oyoshi, T., M. Nakayama, and J. Kuratsu, Relationship between aneurysmal subarachnoid hemorrhage and climatic conditions in the subtropical region, Amami-Oshima, in Japan. *Neurol. Med. Chir.,* (Tokyo), 1999. 39(8): p. 585-90; discussion 590-1.

[39] Buxton, N., et al., Relationship of aneurysmal subarachnoid hemorrhage to changes in atmospheric pressure: results of a prospective study. *J. Neurosurg.*, 2001. 95(3): p. 391-2.

[40] Beseoglu, K., et al., Dependence of subarachnoid hemorrhage on climate conditions: a systematic meteorological analysis from the dusseldorf metropolitan area. *Neurosurgery,* 2008. 62(5): p. 1033-8; discussion 1038-9.

[41] Kaneko, A., et al., Malaria epidemiology, glucose 6-phosphate dehydrogenase deficiency and human settlement in the Vanuatu Archipelago. *Acta. Trop.*, 1998. 70(3): p. 285-302.

[42] Locksley, H. B., Natural history of subarachnoid hemorrhage, intracranial aneurysms and arteriovenous malformations. *J. Neurosurg.,* 1966. 25(3): p. 321-68.

[43] Yasui, N., et al., Subarachnoid hemorrhage caused by previously diagnosed, previously unruptured intracranial aneurysms: a retrospective analysis of 25 cases. *Neurosurgery,* 1996. 39(6): p. 1096-100; discussion 1100-1.

[44] Ferguson, G. G., S. J. Peerless, and C. G. Drake, Natural history of intracranial aneurysms. *N. Engl. J. Med.,* 1981. 305(2): p. 99.

[45] Hsiang, J. N., et al., The role of computed tomographic angiography in the diagnosis of intracranial aneurysms and emergent aneurysm clipping. *Neurosurgery,* 1996. 38(3): p. 481-7 discussion 487.

[46] Sarti, C., et al., Epidemiology of subarachnoid hemorrhage in Finland from 1983 to 1985. *Stroke,* 1991. 22(7): p. 848-53.

[47] Asari, S. and T. Ohmoto, Natural history and risk factors of unruptured cerebral aneurysms. *Clin. Neurol. Neurosurg.,* 1993. 95(3): p. 205-14.

[48] Juvela, S., M. Porras, and O. Heiskanen, Natural history of unruptured intracranial aneurysms: a long-term follow-up study. *J. Neurosurg.,* 1993. 79(2): p. 174-82.

[49] Winn, H. R., et al., The long-term outcome in patients with multiple aneurysms. Incidence of late hemorrhage and implications for treatment of incidental aneurysms. *J. Neurosurg.*, 1983. 59(4): p. 642-51.

[50] Vieco, P. T., et al., Detection of circle of Willis aneurysms in patients with acute subarachnoid hemorrhage: a comparison of CT angiography and digital subtraction angiography. *AJR Am. J. Roentgenol.*, 1995. 165(2): p. 425-30.

[51] King, J. T., Jr., J. A. Berlin, and E. S. Flamm, Morbidity and mortality from elective surgery for asymptomatic, unruptured, intracranial aneurysms: a meta-analysis. *J. Neurosurg.*, 1994. 81(6): p. 837-42.

[52] Raaymakers, T. W., G. J. Rinkel, and L. M. Ramos, Initial and follow-up screening for aneurysms in families with familial subarachnoid hemorrhage. *Neurology*, 1998. 51(4): p. 1125-30.

[53] Ronkainen, A., et al., Risk of harboring an unruptured intracranial aneurysm. *Stroke*, 1998. 29(2): p. 359-62.

[54] Kojima, M., et al., Asymptomatic familial cerebral aneurysms. *Neurosurgery*, 1998. 43(4): p. 776-81.

[55] Zhang, B., et al., Polymorphisms in matrix metalloproteinase-1, -3, -9, and -12 genes in relation to subarachnoid hemorrhage. *Stroke*, 2001. 32(9): p. 2198-202.

[56] Tsutsumi, K., et al., Risk of aneurysm recurrence in patients with clipped cerebral aneurysms: results of long-term follow-up angiography. *Stroke*, 2001. 32(5): p. 1191-4.

[57] Rinne, J. K. and J. A. Hernesniemi, De novo aneurysms: special multiple intracranial aneurysms. *Neurosurgery*, 1993. 33(6): p. 981-5.

[58] Inagawa, T. and A. Hirano, Autopsy study of unruptured incidental intracranial aneurysms. *Surg. Neurol.*, 1990. 34(6): p. 361-5.

[59] Zacks, D. J., D. B. Russell, and J. D. Miller, Fortuitously discovered intracranial aneurysms. *Arch. Neurol.*, 1980. 37(1): p. 39-41.

[60] David, C. A., et al., Late angiographic follow-up review of surgically treated aneurysms. *J. Neurosurg.*, 1999. 91(3): p. 396-401.

[61] Miller, C. A., S. A. Hill, and W. E. Hunt, "De novo" aneurysms. A clinical review. *Surg. Neurol.*, 1985. 24(2): p. 173-80.

[62] Raabe, A., et al., [Recommendations for the management of unruptured intracranial aneurysms]. *Zentralbl. Neurochir.*, 2002. 63(2): p. 70-6.

[63] Bassi, P., et al., Warning signs in subarachnoid hemorrhage: a cooperative study. *Acta. Neurol. Scand.*, 1991. 84(4): p. 277-81.

[64] Weir, B., Antifibrinolytics in subarachnoid hemorrhage. Do they have a role? No. *Arch. Neurol.*, 1987. 44(1): p. 116-8.

[65] Hauerberg, J., et al., Importance of the recognition of a warning leak as a sign of a ruptured intracranial aneurysm. *Acta. Neurol. Scand.*, 1991. 83(1): p. 61-4.
[66] Schievink, W. I., Intracranial aneurysms. *N. Engl. J. Med.*, 1997. 336(1): p. 28-40.
[67] Yano, K., D. M. Reed, and C. J. MacLean, Serum cholesterol and hemorrhagic stroke in the Honolulu Heart Program. *Stroke,* 1989. 20(11): p. 1460-5.
[68] Sundaram, M. B. and F. Chow, Seizures associated with spontaneous subarachnoid hemorrhage. *Can. J. Neurol. Sci.,* 1986. 13(3): p. 229-31.
[69] Kapapa, T. and E. Rickels, Health-related quality of life after subarachnoid hemorrhage. *Neurol. Rehabil.*, 2005. 11(1): p. 21-28.
[70] Korogi, Y., et al., Intracranial aneurysms: detection with three-dimensional CT angiography with volume rendering--comparison with conventional angiographic and surgical findings. *Radiology,* 1999. 211(2): p. 497-506.
[71] Hope, J. K., J. L. Wilson, and F. J. Thomson, Three-dimensional CT angiography in the detection and characterization of intracranial berry aneurysms. *AJNR Am. J. Neuroradiol.*, 1996. 17(3): p. 439-45.
[72] Alberico, R. A., et al., Evaluation of the circle of Willis with three-dimensional CT angiography in patients with suspected intracranial aneurysms. *AJNR Am. J. Neuroradiol.,* 1995. 16(8): p. 1571-8; discussion 1579-80.
[73] Liang, E. Y., et al., Detection and assessment of intracranial aneurysms: value of CT angiography with shaded-surface display. *AJR Am. J. Roentgenol.*, 1995. 165(6): p. 1497-502.
[74] Ogawa, T., et al., Cerebral aneurysms: evaluation with three-dimensional CT angiography. *AJNR Am. J. Neuroradiol.*, 1996. 17(3): p. 447-54.
[75] Wilms, G., et al., Spiral CT of intracranial aneurysms: correlation with digital subtraction and magnetic resonance angiography. *Neuroradiology*, 1996. 38 Suppl. 1: p. S20-5.
[76] Backes, D., et al., Time-dependent test characteristics of head computed tomography in patients suspected of nontraumatic subarachnoid hemorrhage. *Stroke,* 2012. 43(8): p. 2115-9.
[77] Steiner, T., et al., European Stroke Organization guidelines for the management of intracranial aneurysms and subarachnoid hemorrhage. *Cerebrovasc. Dis.*, 2013. 35(2): p. 93-112.

[78] Hodel, J., et al., Double Inversion Recovery MR Sequence for the Detection of Subacute Subarachnoid Hemorrhage. *AJNR Am. J. Neuroradiol.*, 2014.

[79] Huston, J., 3rd, et al., Blinded prospective evaluation of sensitivity of MR angiography to known intracranial aneurysms: importance of aneurysm size. *AJNR Am. J. Neuroradiol.*, 1994. 15(9): p. 1607-14.

[80] Anzalone, N., F. Triulzi, and G. Scotti, Acute subarachnoid hemorrhage: 3D time-of-flight MR angiography versus intra-arterial digital angiography. *Neuroradiology*, 1995. 37(4): p. 257-61.

[81] Atlas, S. W., Magnetic resonance imaging of intracranial aneurysms. *Neuroimaging Clin. N. Am.*, 1997. 7(4): p. 709-20.

[82] Wilcock, D., et al., Comparison of magnetic resonance angiography with conventional angiography in the detection of intracranial aneurysms in patients presenting with subarachnoid hemorrhage. *Clin. Radiol.*, 1996. 51(5): p. 330-4.

[83] Stewart, H., A. Reuben, and J. McDonald, LP or not LP, that is the question: gold standard or unnecessary procedure in subarachnoid hemorrhage? *Emerg. Med. J.*, 2014. 31(9): p. 720-3.

[84] Agid, R., et al., Negative CT angiography findings in patients with spontaneous subarachnoid hemorrhage: When is digital subtraction angiography still needed? *AJNR Am. J. Neuroradiol.*, 2010. 31(4): p. 696-705.

[85] Hunt, W. E. and R. M. Hess, Surgical risk as related to time of intervention in the repair of intracranial aneurysms. *J. Neurosurg.*, 1968. 28(1): p. 14-20.

[86] Fisher, C. M., J. P. Kistler, and J. M. Davis, Relation of cerebral vasospasm to subarachnoid hemorrhage visualized by computerized tomographic scanning. *Neurosurgery,* 1980. 6(1): p. 1-9.

[87] Teasdale, G. and B. Jennett, Assessment of coma and impaired consciousness. A practical scale. *Lancet,* 1974. 2(7872): p. 81-4.

[88] Ogungbo, B., The World Federation of Neurological Surgeons scale for subarachnoid hemorrhage. *Surg. Neurol.,* 2003. 59(3): p. 236-7; discussion 237-8.

[89] Rosen, D. S. and R. L. Macdonald, Subarachnoid hemorrhage grading scales: a systematic review. *Neurocrit. Care,* 2005. 2(2): p. 110-8.

[90] Oshiro, E. M., et al., A new subarachnoid hemorrhage grading system based on the Glasgow Coma Scale: a comparison with the Hunt and Hess and World Federation of Neurological Surgeons Scales in a clinical series. *Neurosurgery,* 1997. 41(1): p. 140-7; discussion 147-8.

[91] Henderson, W. G., J. C. Torner, and D. W. Nibbelink, Intracranial aneurysms and subarachnoid hemorrhage --- report on a randomized treatment study. IV-B. Regulated bed rest --- statistical evaluation. *Stroke,* 1977. 8(5): p. 579-89.
[92] Nibbelink, D. W., J. C. Torner, and W. G. Henderson, Intracranial aneurysms and subarachnoid hemorrhage - report on a randomized treatment study. IV-A. regulated bed rest. *Stroke,* 1977. 8(2): p. 202-18.
[93] Adams, H. P., Jr., et al., Antifibrinolytic therapy in patients with aneurysmal subarachnoid hemorrhage. A report of the cooperative aneurysm study. *Arch. Neurol.,* 1981. 38(1): p. 25-9.
[94] Nishioka, H., et al., Cooperative study of intracranial aneurysms and subarachnoid hemorrhage: a long-term prognostic study. III. Subarachnoid hemorrhage of undetermined etiology. *Arch. Neurol.,* 1984. 41(11): p. 1147-51.
[95] Kassell, N. F., et al., Overall management of ruptured aneurysm: comparison of early and late operation. *Neurosurgery,* 1981. 9(2): p. 120-8.
[96] Nishioka, H., et al., Cooperative study of intracranial aneurysms and subarachnoid hemorrhage: a long-term prognostic study. II. Ruptured intracranial aneurysms managed conservatively. *Arch. Neurol.,* 1984. 41(11): p. 1142-6.
[97] Auer, L. M., Unfavorable outcome following early surgical repair of ruptured cerebral aneurysms--a critical review of 238 patients. *Surg. Neurol.*, 1991. 35(2): p. 152-8.
[98] Kassell, N. F. and C. G. Drake, Timing of aneurysm surgery. *Neurosurgery*, 1982. 10(4): p. 514-9.
[99] Kassell, N. F. and J. C. Torner, The International Cooperative study on timing of aneurysm surgery. *Acta. Neurochir.*, (Wien), 1982. 63(1-4): p. 119-23.
[100] Chyatte, D., N. C. Fode, and T. M. Sundt, Jr., Early versus late intracranial aneurysm surgery in subarachnoid hemorrhage. *J. Neurosurg.,* 1988. 69(3): p. 326-31.
[101] Ohman, J. and O. Heiskanen, Timing of operation for ruptured supratentorial aneurysms: a prospective randomized study. *J. Neurosurg.*, 1989. 70(1): p. 55-60.
[102] Ohkuma, H., H. Tsurutani, and S. Suzuki, Incidence and significance of early aneurysmal rebleeding before neurosurgical or neurological management. *Stroke*, 2001. 32(5): p. 1176-80.

[103] Fujii, Y., et al., Ultra-early rebleeding in spontaneous subarachnoid hemorrhage. *J. Neurosurg.,* 1996. 84(1): p. 35-42.
[104] Adams, H. P., Jr., Early management of the patient with recent aneurysmal subarachnoid hemorrhage. *Stroke,* 1986. 17(6): p. 1068-70.
[105] Adams, H. P., Jr., et al., Early management of aneurysmal subarachnoid hemorrhage. A report of the Cooperative Aneurysm Study. *J. Neurosurg.*, 1981. 54(2): p. 141-5.
[106] Guglielmi, G., et al., Electrothrombosis of saccular aneurysms via endovascular approach. Part 2: Preliminary clinical experience. *J. Neurosurg.*, 1991. 75(1): p. 8-14.
[107] Guglielmi, G., et al., Electrothrombosis of saccular aneurysms via endovascular approach. Part 1: Electrochemical basis, technique, and experimental results. *J. Neurosurg.,* 1991. 75(1): p. 1-7.
[108] Guglielmi, G., History of the genesis of detachable coils. A review. *J. Neurosurg.,* 2009. 111(1): p. 1-8.
[109] Guglielmi, G., History of detachable coils: the backdrop. *J. Neurosurg.*, 2010. 112(1): p. 217-8.
[110] Hui, F. K., et al., A history of detachable coils: 1987-2012. *J. Neurointerv. Surg*., 2014. 6(2): p. 134-8.
[111] Brilstra, E. H., et al., Treatment of intracranial aneurysms by embolization with coils: a systematic review. *Stroke,* 1999. 30(2): p. 470-6.
[112] Bejjani, G. K., et al., The efficacy and safety of angioplasty for cerebral vasospasm after subarachnoid hemorrhage. *Neurosurgery,* 1998. 42(5): p. 979-86; discussion 986-7.
[113] Molyneux, A. J., et al., International subarachnoid aneurysm trial (ISAT) of neurosurgical clipping versus endovascular coiling in 2143 patients with ruptured intracranial aneurysms: a randomised comparison of effects on survival, dependency, seizures, rebleeding, subgroups, and aneurysm occlusion. *Lancet,* 2005. 366(9488): p. 809-17.
[114] Wiebers, D. O., et al., Unruptured intracranial aneurysms: natural history, clinical outcome, and risks of surgical and endovascular treatment. *Lancet,* 2003. 362(9378): p. 103-10.
[115] Cognard, C., et al., Long-term angiographic follow-up of 169 intracranial berry aneurysms occluded with detachable coils. *Radiology,* 1999. 212(2): p. 348-56.
[116] Koivisto, T., et al., Outcomes of early endovascular versus surgical treatment of ruptured cerebral aneurysms. A prospective randomized study. *Stroke*, 2000. 31(10): p. 2369-77.

[117] Byrne, J. V., Long-term outcomes of Guglielmi detachable coil packing for acutely ruptured cerebral aneurysms. *AJNR Am. J. Neuroradiol.*, 1999. 20(6): p. 1184.
[118] Cognard, C., et al., Intracranial berry aneurysms: angiographic and clinical results after endovascular treatment. *Radiology*, 1998. 206(2): p. 499-510.
[119] Uda, K., et al., Embolization of cerebral aneurysms using Guglielmi detachable coils--problems and treatment plans in the acute stage after subarachnoid hemorrhage and long-term efficiency. *Neurol. Med. Chir.*, (Tokyo), 1998. 38(3): p. 143-52; discussion 152-4.
[120] Graves, V. B., et al., Early treatment of ruptured aneurysms with Guglielmi detachable coils: effect on subsequent bleeding. *Neurosurgery*, 1995. 37(4): p. 640-7; discussion 647-8.
[121] Casasco, A. E., et al., Selective endovascular treatment of 71 intracranial aneurysms with platinum coils. *J. Neurosurg.*, 1993. 79(1): p. 3-10.
[122] Sluzewski, M. and W. J. van Rooij, Early rebleeding after coiling of ruptured cerebral aneurysms: incidence, morbidity, and risk factors. *AJNR Am. J. Neuroradiol.*, 2005. 26(7): p. 1739-43.
[123] Byrne, J. V., et al., Five-year experience in using coil embolization for ruptured intracranial aneurysms: outcomes and incidence of late rebleeding. *J. Neurosurg.*, 1999. 90(4): p. 656-63.
[124] Hayakawa, M., et al., Natural history of the neck remnant of a cerebral aneurysm treated with the Guglielmi detachable coil system. *J. Neurosurg.*, 2000. 93(4): p. 561-8.
[125] Rates of delayed rebleeding from intracranial aneurysms are low after surgical and endovascular treatment. *Stroke*, 2006. 37(6): p. 1437-42.
[126] Murayama, Y., et al., Guglielmi detachable coil embolization of cerebral aneurysms: 11 years' experience. *J. Neurosurg.*, 2003. 98(5): p. 959-66.
[127] Johnston, S. C., et al., Surgical and endovascular treatment of unruptured cerebral aneurysms at university hospitals. *Neurology*, 1999. 52(9): p. 1799-805.
[128] Raftopoulos, C., et al., Prospective analysis of aneurysm treatment in a series of 103 consecutive patients when endovascular embolization is considered the first option. *J. Neurosurg.*, 2000. 93(2): p. 175-82.
[129] Regli, L., et al., Endovascular coiling compared with surgical clipping for the treatment of unruptured middle cerebral artery aneurysms: an update. *Acta. Neurochir. Suppl.*, 2002. 82: p. 41-6.
[130] Regli, L., A. Uske, and N. de Tribolet, Endovascular coil placement compared with surgical clipping for the treatment of unruptured middle

cerebral artery aneurysms: a consecutive series. *J. Neurosurg.,* 1999. 90(6): p. 1025-30.

[131] Suzuki, J., T. Yoshimoto, and T. Kayama, Surgical treatment of middle cerebral artery aneurysms. *J. Neurosurg.*, 1984. 61(1): p. 17-23.

[132] Khanna, R. K., G. M. Malik, and N. Qureshi, Predicting outcome following surgical treatment of unruptured intracranial aneurysms: a proposed grading system. *J. Neurosurg.,* 1996. 84(1): p. 49-54.

[133] Rinne, J., et al., Analysis of 561 patients with 690 middle cerebral artery aneurysms: anatomic and clinical features as correlated to management outcome. *Neurosurgery,* 1996. 38(1): p. 2-11.

[134] Johnston, S. C., et al., Endovascular and surgical treatment of unruptured cerebral aneurysms: comparison of risks. *Ann. Neurol.,* 2000. 48(1): p. 11-9.

[135] Gruber, D. P., et al., A comparison between endovascular and surgical management of basilar artery apex aneurysms. *J. Neurosurg.,* 1999. 90(5): p. 868-74.

[136] Halbach, V. V., et al., Cavernous internal carotid artery aneurysms treated with electrolytically detachable coils. *J. Neuroophthalmol.*, 1997. 17(4): p. 231-9.

[137] Halbach, V. V., et al., The efficacy of endosaccular aneurysm occlusion in alleviating neurological deficits produced by mass effect. *J. Neurosurg.*, 1994. 80(4): p. 659-66.

[138] Yundt, K. D., et al., Cerebral hemodynamic and metabolic changes caused by brain retraction after aneurysmal subarachnoid hemorrhage. *Neurosurgery*, 1997. 40(3): p. 442-50; discussion 450-1.

[139] Kremer, C., et al., Outcome after endovascular treatment of Hunt and Hess grade IV or V aneurysms: comparison of anterior versus posterior circulation. *Stroke,* 1999. 30(12): p. 2617-22.

[140] Feuerberg, I., et al., Natural history of postoperative aneurysm rests. *J. Neurosurg.,* 1987. 66(1): p. 30-4.

[141] Hop, J. W., et al., Case-fatality rates and functional outcome after subarachnoid hemorrhage: a systematic review. *Stroke,* 1997. 28(3): p. 660-4.

[142] Gross, B. A., et al., Treatment Modality and Vasospasm After Aneurysmal Subarachnoid Hemorrhage. *World Neurosurg.*, 2013.

[143] Al-Tamimi, Y. Z., et al., A review of delayed ischemic neurologic deficit following aneurysmal subarachnoid hemorrhage: historical overview, current treatment, and pathophysiology. *World Neurosurg.,* 2010. 73(6): p. 654-67.

[144] Dorsch, N., A clinical review of cerebral vasospasm and delayed ischaemia following aneurysm rupture. *Acta. Neurochir. Suppl.,* 2011. 110(Pt 1): p. 5-6.
[145] Washington, C. W., G. J. Zipfel, and H. Participants in the International Multi-disciplinary Consensus Conference on the Critical Care Management of Subarachnoid, Detection and monitoring of vasospasm and delayed cerebral ischemia: a review and assessment of the literature. *Neurocrit. Care,* 2011. 15(2): p. 312-7.
[146] Chalouhi, N., et al., Endovascular management of cerebral vasospasm following aneurysm rupture: outcomes and predictors in 116 patients. *Clin. Neurol. Neurosurg.,* 2014. 118: p. 26-31.
[147] Hayashi, K., et al., Current status of endovascular treatment for vasospasm following subarachnoid hemorrhage: analysis of JR-NET2. *Neurol. Med. Chir.,* (Tokyo), 2014. 54(2): p. 107-12.
[148] Heros, R. C., N. T. Zervas, and V. Varsos, Cerebral vasospasm after subarachnoid hemorrhage: an update. *Ann. Neurol.,* 1983. 14(6): p. 599-608.
[149] Fisher, C. M., G. H. Roberson, and R.G. Ojemann, Cerebral vasospasm with ruptured saccular aneurysm--the clinical manifestations. *Neurosurgery,* 1977. 1(3): p. 245-8.
[150] Haley, E. C., Jr., N. F. Kassell, and J. C. Torner, The International Cooperative Study on the Timing of Aneurysm Surgery. The North American experience. *Stroke,* 1992. 23(2): p. 205-14.
[151] Longstreth, W. T., Jr., et al., Clinical course of spontaneous subarachnoid hemorrhage: a population-based study in King County, Washington. *Neurology,* 1993. 43(4): p. 712-8.
[152] Aaslid, R., P. Huber, and H. Nornes, Evaluation of cerebrovascular spasm with transcranial Doppler ultrasound. *J. Neurosurg.,* 1984. 60(1): p. 37-41.
[153] Aaslid, R., T. M. Markwalder, and H. Nornes, Noninvasive transcranial Doppler ultrasound recording of flow velocity in basal cerebral arteries. *J. Neurosurg.,* 1982. 57(6): p. 769-74.
[154] Aaslid, R., P. Huber, and H. Nornes, A transcranial Doppler method in the evaluation of cerebrovascular spasm. *Neuroradiology,* 1986. 28(1): p. 11-6.
[155] Ekelund, A., et al., Is transcranial Doppler sonography useful in detecting late cerebral ischaemia after aneurysmal subarachnoid hemorrhage? *Br. J. Neurosurg.,* 1996. 10(1): p. 19-25.

[156] Grosset, D. G., et al., Prediction of symptomatic vasospasm after subarachnoid hemorrhage by rapidly increasing transcranial Doppler velocity and cerebral blood flow changes. *Stroke,* 1992. 23(5): p. 674-9.

[157] Lindegaard, K. F., et al., Cerebral vasospasm diagnosis by means of angiography and blood velocity measurements. *Acta. Neurochir.,* (Wien), 1989. 100(1-2): p. 12-24.

[158] Vora, Y. Y., et al., Role of transcranial Doppler monitoring in the diagnosis of cerebral vasospasm after subarachnoid hemorrhage. *Neurosurgery,* 1999. 44(6): p. 1237-47; discussion 1247-8.

[159] Sloan, M. A., et al., Assessment: transcranial Doppler ultrasonography: report of the Therapeutics and Technology Assessment Subcommittee of the American Academy of Neurology. *Neurology,* 2004. 62(9): p. 1468-81.

[160] Sloan, M. A., et al., Sensitivity and specificity of transcranial Doppler ultrasonography in the diagnosis of vasospasm following subarachnoid hemorrhage. *Neurology,* 1989. 39(11): p. 1514-8.

[161] Solomon, R. A., M. E. Fink, and L. Lennihan, Early aneurysm surgery and prophylactic hypervolemic hypertensive therapy for the treatment of aneurysmal subarachnoid hemorrhage. *Neurosurgery,* 1988. 23(6): p. 699-704.

[162] Mayberg, M. R., et al., Guidelines for the management of aneurysmal subarachnoid hemorrhage. A statement for healthcare professionals from a special writing group of the Stroke Council, American Heart Association. *Circulation*, 1994. 90(5): p. 2592-605.

[163] Allen, G. S., et al., Cerebral arterial spasm--a controlled trial of nimodipine in patients with subarachnoid hemorrhage. *N. Engl. J. Med.,* 1983. 308(11): p. 619-24.

[164] Haley, E. C., Jr., et al., A randomized trial of two doses of nicardipine in aneurysmal subarachnoid hemorrhage. A report of the Cooperative Aneurysm Study. *J. Neurosurg.*, 1994. 80(5): p. 788-96.

[165] Barth, M., et al., Effect of nicardipine prolonged-release implants on cerebral vasospasm and clinical outcome after severe aneurysmal subarachnoid hemorrhage: a prospective, randomized, double-blind phase IIa study. *Stroke,* 2007. 38(2): p. 330-6.

[166] Dorhout Mees, S. M., et al., Calcium antagonists for aneurysmal subarachnoid hemorrhage. *Cochrane Database Syst. Rev.*, 2007(3): p. CD000277.

[167] Dorhout Mees, S. M., et al., Calcium Antagonists for Aneurysmal Subarachnoid Hemorrhage. *Stroke,* 2008.

[168] van den Bergh, W. M., et al., Randomized controlled trial of acetylsalicylic acid in aneurysmal subarachnoid hemorrhage: the MASH Study. *Stroke,* 2006. 37(9): p. 2326-30.

[169] Hop, J. W., et al., Randomized pilot trial of postoperative aspirin in subarachnoid hemorrhage. *Neurology,* 2000. 54(4): p. 872-8.

[170] Lanzino, G., et al., Double-blind, randomized, vehicle-controlled study of high-dose tirilazad mesylate in women with aneurysmal subarachnoid hemorrhage. Part I. A cooperative study in Europe, Australia, New Zealand, and South Africa. *J. Neurosurg.*, 1999. 90(6): p. 1011-7.

[171] Lanzino, G. and N. F. Kassell, Double-blind, randomized, vehicle-controlled study of high-dose tirilazad mesylate in women with aneurysmal subarachnoid hemorrhage. Part II. A cooperative study in North America. *J. Neurosurg.*, 1999. 90(6): p. 1018-24.

[172] Asano, T., et al., Effects of a hydroxyl radical scavenger on delayed ischemic neurological deficits following aneurysmal subarachnoid hemorrhage: results of a multicenter, placebo-controlled double-blind trial. *J. Neurosurg.,* 1996. 84(5): p. 792-803.

[173] Haley, E. C., Jr., et al., A randomized, double-blind, vehicle-controlled trial of tirilazad mesylate in patients with aneurysmal subarachnoid hemorrhage: a cooperative study in North America. *J. Neurosurg.*, 1997. 86(3): p. 467-74.

[174] Kassell, N. F., et al., Randomized, double-blind, vehicle-controlled trial of tirilazad mesylate in patients with aneurysmal subarachnoid hemorrhage: a cooperative study in Europe, Australia, and New Zealand. *J. Neurosurg.,* 1996. 84(2): p. 221-8.

[175] Lynch, J. R., et al., Simvastatin reduces vasospasm after aneurysmal subarachnoid hemorrhage: results of a pilot randomized clinical trial. *Stroke,* 2005. 36(9): p. 2024-6.

[176] Reinert, M., et al., Transdermal nitroglycerin in patients with subarachnoid hemorrhage. *Neurol. Res.*, 2004. 26(4): p. 435-9.

[177] Saito, I., et al., Neuroprotective effect of an antioxidant, ebselen, in patients with delayed neurological deficits after aneurysmal subarachnoid hemorrhage. *Neurosurgery,* 1998. 42(2): p. 269-77; discussion 277-8.

[178] Shaw, M. D., et al., Efficacy and safety of the endothelin, receptor antagonist TAK-044 in treating subarachnoid hemorrhage: a report by the Steering Committee on behalf of the UK/Netherlands/Eire TAK-044 Subarachnoid Hemorrhage Study Group. *J. Neurosurg.*, 2000. 93(6): p. 992-7.

[179] Tseng, M. Y., et al., Effects of acute treatment with pravastatin on cerebral vasospasm, autoregulation, and delayed ischemic deficits after aneurysmal subarachnoid hemorrhage: a phase II randomized placebo-controlled trial. *Stroke,* 2005. 36(8): p. 1627-32.
[180] Vajkoczy, P., et al., Clazosentan (AXV-034343), a selective endothelin A receptor antagonist, in the prevention of cerebral vasospasm following severe aneurysmal subarachnoid hemorrhage: results of a randomized, double-blind, placebo-controlled, multicenter phase IIa study. *J. Neurosurg.,* 2005. 103(1): p. 9-17.
[181] Johnston, S. C., Effect of endovascular services and hospital volume on cerebral aneurysm treatment outcomes. *Stroke,* 2000. 31(1): p. 111-7.
[182] Eskridge, J. M. and J. K. Song, Endovascular embolization of 150 basilar tip aneurysms with Guglielmi detachable coils: results of the Food and Drug Administration multicenter clinical trial. *J. Neurosurg.,* 1998. 89(1): p. 81-6.
[183] Eskridge, J. M. and J. K. Song, A practical approach to the treatment of vasospasm. *AJNR Am. J. Neuroradiol.,* 1997. 18(9): p. 1653-60.
[184] Eskridge, J. M., D. W. Newell, and H. R. Winn, Endovascular treatment of vasospasm. *Neurosurg. Clin. N. Am.,* 1994. 5(3): p. 437-47.
[185] Zubkov, Y. N., B. M. Nikiforov, and V. A. Shustin, Balloon catheter technique for dilatation of constricted cerebral arteries after aneurysmal SAH. *Acta. Neurochir.,* (Wien), 1984. 70(1-2): p. 65-79.
[186] Newell, D. W., et al., Angioplasty for the treatment of symptomatic vasospasm following subarachnoid hemorrhage. *J. Neurosurg.,* 1989. 71(5 Pt 1): p. 654-60.
[187] Cross, D. T., 3rd, et al., Intracranial pressure monitoring during intraarterial papaverine infusion for cerebral vasospasm. *AJNR Am. J. Neuroradiol.,* 1998. 19(7): p. 1319-23.
[188] Mathis, J. M., M. E. Jensen, and J. E. Dion, Technical considerations on intra-arterial papaverine hydrochloride for cerebral vasospasm. *Neuroradiology,* 1997. 39(2): p. 90-8.
[189] McAuliffe, W., et al., Intracranial pressure changes induced during papaverine infusion for treatment of vasospasm. *J. Neurosurg.,* 1995. 83(3): p. 430-4.
[190] Milburn, J. M., et al., Effect of intraarterial papaverine on cerebral circulation time. *AJNR Am. J. Neuroradiol.,* 1997. 18(6): p. 1081-5.
[191] Clyde, B. L., et al., Paradoxical aggravation of vasospasm with papaverine infusion following aneurysmal subarachnoid hemorrhage. Case report. *J. Neurosurg.,* 1996. 84(4): p. 690-5.

[192] Coyne, T. J., et al., Percutaneous transluminal angioplasty for cerebral vasospasm after subarachnoid hemorrhage. *Can. J. Surg.,* 1994. 37(5): p. 391-6.

[193] Elliott, J. P., et al., Comparison of balloon angioplasty and papaverine infusion for the treatment of vasospasm following aneurysmal subarachnoid hemorrhage. *J. Neurosurg.,* 1998. 88(2): p. 277-84.

[194] Beck, J., et al., Perfusion-weighted magnetic resonance imaging in patients with vasospasm: a useful new tool in the management of patients with subarachnoid hemorrhage. *Neurosurgery,* 2006. 58(3): p. E590; author reply E590.

[195] Otawara, Y., et al., Evaluation of vasospasm after subarachnoid hemorrhage by use of multislice computed tomographic angiography. *Neurosurgery,* 2002. 51(4): p. 939-42; discussion 942-3.

[196] Turowski, B., et al., [Cerebral perfusion computerized tomography in vasospasm after subarachnoid hemorrhage: diagnostic value of MTT]. *Rofo,* 2007. 179(8): p. 847-54.

[197] Weidauer, S., et al., Impairment of cerebral perfusion and infarct patterns attributable to vasospasm after aneurysmal subarachnoid hemorrhage: a prospective MRI and DSA study. *Stroke,* 2007. 38(6): p. 1831-6.

[198] Lai, L. and M. K. Morgan, Predictors of in-hospital shunt-dependent hydrocephalus following rupture of cerebral aneurysms. *J. Clin. Neurosci.,* 2013. 20(8): p. 1134-8.

[199] Fugate, J. E., et al., Aggressive CSF diversion reverses delayed cerebral ischemia in aneurysmal subarachnoid hemorrhage: a case report. *Neurocrit. Care,* 2012. 17(1): p. 112-6.

[200] Della Pepa, G. M., et al., Protective effect of external ventricular drainage on cerebral vasospasm. A retrospective study on aneurysmal SAH treated endovascularly. *Clin. Neurol. Neurosurg.,* 2014. 124: p. 97-101.

[201] Butzkueven, H., et al., Onset seizures independently predict poor outcome after subarachnoid hemorrhage. *Neurology,* 2000. 55(9): p. 1315-20.

[202] Lin, C. L., et al., Characterization of perioperative seizures and epilepsy following aneurysmal subarachnoid hemorrhage. *J. Neurosurg.,* 2003. 99(6): p. 978-85.

[203] Rhoney, D. H., et al., Anticonvulsant prophylaxis and timing of seizures after aneurysmal subarachnoid hemorrhage. *Neurology,* 2000. 55(2): p. 258-65.

[204] Claassen, J., et al., Predictors and clinical impact of epilepsy after subarachnoid hemorrhage. *Neurology,* 2003. 60(2): p. 208-14.

[205] Rose, F. C. and M. Sarner, Epilepsy after Ruptured Intracranial Aneurysm. *Br. Med. J.,* 1965. 1(5426): p. 18-21.

[206] Ukkola, V. and E. R. Heikkinen, Epilepsy after operative treatment of ruptured cerebral aneurysms. *Acta. Neurochir.*, (Wien), 1990. 106(3-4): p. 115-8.

[207] Kvam, D. A., et al., Seizures during the immediate postoperative period. *Neurosurgery,* 1983. 12(1): p. 14-7.

[208] Cabral, R. J., T. T. King, and D. F. Scott, Epilepsy after two different neurosurgical approaches to the treatment of ruptured intracranial aneurysm. *J. Neurol. Neurosurg. Psychiatry,* 1976. 39(11): p. 1052-6.

[209] Kotila, M. and O. Waltimo, Epilepsy after stroke. *Epilepsia,* 1992. 33(3): p. 495-8.

[210] Ohman, J., Hypertension as a risk factor for epilepsy after aneurysmal subarachnoid hemorrhage and surgery. *Neurosurgery,* 1990. 27(4): p. 578-81.

[211] Hart, R. G., et al., Occurrence and implications of seizures in subarachnoid hemorrhage due to ruptured intracranial aneurysms. *Neurosurgery,* 1981. 8(4): p. 417-21.

[212] Naidech, A. M., et al., Phenytoin exposure is associated with functional and cognitive disability after subarachnoid hemorrhage. *Stroke,* 2005. 36(3): p. 583-7.

[213] O'Laoire, S. A., Epilepsy following neurosurgical intervention. *Acta. Neurochir. Suppl.,* (Wien), 1990. 50: p. 52-4.

[214] Mak, C. H., Y. Y. Lu, and G. K. Wong, Review and recommendations on management of refractory raised intracranial pressure in aneurysmal subarachnoid hemorrhage. *Vasc. Health Risk Manag.*, 2013. 9: p. 353-9.

[215] Otani, N., et al., Surgical results after primary decompressive craniectomy in poor-grade aneurysmal subarachnoid hemorrhage. *Acta. Neurochir. Suppl.*, 2013. 118: p. 269-72.

[216] Uozumi, Y., et al., Decompressive craniectomy in patients with aneurysmal subarachnoid hemorrhage: a single-center matched-pair analysis. *Cerebrovasc. Dis.*, 2014. 37(2): p. 109-15.

[217] D'Ambrosio, A. L., et al., Decompressive hemicraniectomy for poor-grade aneurysmal subarachnoid hemorrhage patients with associated intracerebral hemorrhage: clinical outcome and quality of life assessment. *Neurosurgery,* 2005. 56(1): p. 12-9; dicussion 19-20.

[218] Otani, N., et al., Surgical outcome following decompressive craniectomy for poor-grade aneurysmal subarachnoid hemorrhage in patients with associated massive intracerebral or Sylvian hematomas. *Cerebrovasc. Dis.*, 2008. 26(6): p. 612-7.
[219] Schirmer, C. M., D. A. Hoit, and A. M. Malek, Decompressive hemicraniectomy for the treatment of intractable intracranial hypertension after aneurysmal subarachnoid hemorrhage. *Stroke,* 2007. 38(3): p. 987-92.
[220] Schievink, W. I., et al., The poor prognosis of ruptured intracranial aneurysms of the posterior circulation. *J. Neurosurg.,* 1995. 82(5): p. 791-5.
[221] Berman, M. F., et al., Impact of hospital-related factors on outcome after treatment of cerebral aneurysms. *Stroke,* 2003. 34(9): p. 2200-7.
[222] van Gijn, J. and K. J. van Dongen, Computed tomography in the diagnosis of subarachnoid hemorrhage and ruptured aneurysm. *Clin. Neurol. Neurosurg.,* 1980. 82(1): p. 11-24.
[223] Yasargil, M. G. and J. L. Fox, The microsurgical approach to intracranial aneurysms. *Surg. Neurol.*, 1975. 3(1): p. 7-14.
[224] Pickard, J. D., et al., Effect of oral nimodipine on cerebral infarction and outcome after subarachnoid hemorrhage: British aneurysm nimodipine trial. *BMJ,* 1989. 298(6674): p. 636-42.
[225] Fogelholm, R., J. Hernesniemi, and M. Vapalahti, Impact of early surgery on outcome after aneurysmal subarachnoid hemorrhage. A population-based study. *Stroke,* 1993. 24(11): p. 1649-54.
[226] Locksley, H. B., Natural history of subarachnoid hemorrhage, intracranial aneurysms and arteriovenous malformations. Based on 6368 cases in the cooperative study. *J. Neurosurg.,* 1966. 25(2): p. 219-39.
[227] Bardach, N. S., et al., Association between subarachnoid hemorrhage outcomes and number of cases treated at California hospitals. *Stroke,* 2002. 33(7): p. 1851-6.
[228] Jennett, B. and M. Bond, Assessment of outcome after severe brain damage. *Lancet,* 1975. 1(7905): p. 480-4.
[229] Rankin, J., Cerebral vascular accidents in patients over the age of 60. II. Prognosis. *Scott. Med. J.*, 1957. 2(5): p. 200-15.
[230] van Swieten, J. C., et al., Interobserver agreement for the assessment of handicap in stroke patients. *Stroke*, 1988. 19(5): p. 604-7.
[231] Seule, M. A., et al., [Aneurysmal subarachnoid hemorrhage - therapy and complications]. *Anasthesiol. Intensivmed. Notfallmed Schmerzther,* 2010. 45(1): p. 8-17.

[232] Hutter, B. O. and J. M. Gilsbach, Which neuropsychological deficits are hidden behind a good outcome (Glasgow = I) after aneurysmal subarachnoid hemorrhage? *Neurosurgery,* 1993. 33(6): p. 999-1006.

[233] Hutter, B. O., J. M. Gilsbach, and I. Kreitschmann, Quality of life and cognitive deficits after subarachnoid hemorrhage. *Br. J. Neurosurg.,* 1995. 9(4): p. 465-475.

[234] Kapapa, T., et al., Healt-related quality of life as amendment to clinical outcome in neurosurgery. *Neurol. Rehabil.*, 2006. 12(1): p. 37-41.

[235] Hutter, B. O., Psychologic adjustment in patients after subarachnoid hemorrhage. *Neuropsychiatry Neuropsychol. Behav. Neurol.,* 1998. 11(1): p. 22-30.

[236] Hutter, B. O. and J. M. Gilsbach, Cognitive deficits after rupture and early repair of anterior communicating artery aneurysms. *Acta. Neurochir.,* (Wien), 1992. 116(1): p. 6-13.

[237] Hutter, B. O. and J. M. Gilsbach, Which neuropsychological deficits are hidden behind a good outcome (Glasgow = I) after aneurysmal subarachnoid hemorrhage? *Neurosurgery,* 1993. 33(6): p. 999-1005; discussion 1005-6.

[238] Hutter, B. O. and J. M. Gilsbach, Early neuropsychological sequelae of aneurysm surgery and subarachnoid hemorrhage. *Acta. Neurochir.,* (Wien), 1996. 138(12): p. 1370-8; discussion 1378-9.

[239] Hutter, B. O., J. M. Gilsbach, and I. Kreitschmann, Is there a difference in cognitive deficits after aneurysmal subarachnoid hemorrhage and subarachnoid hemorrhage of unknown origin? *Acta. Neurochir.,* (Wien), 1994. 127(3-4): p. 129-35.

[240] Hutter, B. O., I. Kreitschmann-Andermahr, and J. M. Gilsbach, Cognitive deficits in the acute stage after subarachnoid hemorrhage. *Neurosurgery,* 1998. 43(5): p. 1054-65.

[241] Hutter, B. O., J. M. Gilsbach, and I. Kreitschmann, Quality of life and cognitive deficits after subarachnoid hemorrhage. *Br. J. Neurosurg.,* 1995. 9(4): p. 465-75.

[242] Perea Bartolome, M. V., V. Ladera Fernandez, and A. Maillo Sanchez, [Long-term cognitive deficits in patients operated on for cerebral aneurysm by craniotomy and clipping]. *Neurologia,* 2009. 24(6): p. 379-85.

[243] Samra, S. K., et al., Recovery of cognitive function after surgery for aneurysmal subarachnoid hemorrhage. *Stroke,* 2007. 38(6): p. 1864-72.

[244] Hutter, B. O., et al., Functional outcome after aneurysmal subarachnoid hemorrhage. *Acta. Neurochir. Suppl.,* 1999. 72: p. 157-74.

[245] Scott, R. B., et al., From multidimensional neuropsychological outcomes to a cognitive complication rate: the International Subarachnoid Aneurysm Trial. *Trials,* 2008. 9: p. 13.
[246] Haug, T., et al., Cognitive outcome after aneurysmal subarachnoid hemorrhage: time course of recovery and relationship to clinical, radiological, and management parameters. *Neurosurgery*, 2007. 60(4): p. 649-56; discussion 656-7.
[247] Kreiter, K. T., et al., Predictors of cognitive dysfunction after subarachnoid hemorrhage. *Stroke,* 2002. 33(1): p. 200-8.
[248] Mayer, S. A., et al., Global and domain-specific cognitive impairment and outcome after subarachnoid hemorrhage. *Neurology,* 2002. 59(11): p. 1750-8.
[249] Hadjivassiliou, M., et al., Aneurysmal SAH: cognitive outcome and structural damage after clipping or coiling. *Neurology,* 2001. 56(12): p. 1672-7.
[250] Tidswell, P., et al., Cognitive outcome after aneurysm rupture: relationship to aneurysm site and perioperative complications. *Neurology,* 1995. 45(5): p. 875-82.
[251] Bornstein, R. A., et al., Neuropsychological function in patients after subarachnoid hemorrhage. *Neurosurgery,* 1987. 21(5): p. 651-4.
[252] Ljunggren, B., et al., Cognitive impairment and adjustment in patients without neurological deficits after aneurysmal SAH and early operation. *J. Neurosurg.,* 1985. 62(5): p. 673-9.
[253] Laiacona, M., et al., Neuropsychological follow-up of patients operated for aneurysms of anterior communicating artery. *Cortex,* 1989. 25(2): p. 261-73.
[254] Brand, C., et al., Cognitive performance following spontaneous subarachnoid hemorrhage versus other forms of intracranial haemorrhage. *Br. J. Neurosurg.*, 2014. 28(1): p. 68-80.
[255] Logue, V., et al., The quality of survival after rupture of an anterior cerebral aneurysm. *Br. J. Psychiatry,* 1968. 114(507): p. 137-60.
[256] Brilstra, E. H., J. W. Hop, and G. J. Rinkel, Quality of life after perimesencephalic haemorrhage. *J. Neurol. Neurosurg. Psychiatry,* 1997. 63(3): p. 382-4.
[257] Hop, J. W., et al., Quality of life in patients and partners after aneurysmal subarachnoid hemorrhage. *Stroke,* 1998. 29(4): p. 798-804.
[258] Hohlrieder, M., et al., Cerebral vasospasm and ischaemic infarction in clipped and coiled intracranial aneurysm patients. *Eur. J. Neurol.,* 2002. 9(4): p. 389-99.

[259] Murayama, Y., et al., Incidence of cerebral vasospasm after endovascular treatment of acutely ruptured aneurysms: report on 69 cases. *J. Neurosurg.,* 1997. 87(6): p. 830-5.

[260] Rabinstein, A. A., et al., Patterns of cerebral infarction in aneurysmal subarachnoid hemorrhage. *Stroke,* 2005. 36(5): p. 992-7.

[261] Yalamanchili, K., et al., Frequency of cerebral vasospasm in patients treated with endovascular occlusion of intracranial aneurysms. *AJNR Am. J. Neuroradiol.,* 1998. 19(3): p. 553-8.

[262] Hutter, B. O., I. Kreitschmann-Andermahr, and J. M. Gilsbach, Health-related quality of life after aneurysmal subarachnoid hemorrhage: impacts of bleeding severity, computerized tomography findings, surgery, vasospasm, and neurological grade. *J. Neurosurg.*, 2001. 94(2): p. 241-51.

[263] Ahola, K., J. Vilkki, and A. Servo, Frontal tests do not detect frontal infarctions after ruptured intracranial aneurysm. *Brain Cogn.,* 1996. 31(1): p. 1-16.

[264] Berry, E., et al., Outcome of subarachnoid hemorrhage. An analysis of surgical variables, cognitive and emotional sequelae related to SPECT scanning. *Br. J. Neurosurg.*, 1997. 11(5): p. 378-87.

[265] Ogden, J. A., T. Utley, and E. W. Mee, Neurological and psychosocial outcome 4 to 7 years after subarachnoid hemorrhage. *Neurosurgery,* 1997. 41(1): p. 25-34.

[266] Sonesson, B., et al., Cognitive functioning after subarachnoid hemorrhage of unknown origin. *Acta. Neurol. Scand.*, 1989. 80(5): p. 400-10.

[267] Vilkki, J. S., et al., Relationship of local infarctions to cognitive and psychosocial impairments after aneurysmal subarachnoid hemorrhage. *Neurosurgery,* 2004. 55(4): p. 790-802; discussion 802-3.

[268] Vilkki, J., et al., Cognitive deficits related to computed tomographic findings after surgery for a ruptured intracranial aneurysm. *Neurosurgery,* 1989. 25(2): p. 166-72.

[269] Kress, J. P., et al., Daily interruption of sedative infusions in critically ill patients undergoing mechanical ventilation. *N. Engl. J. Med.*, 2000. 342(20): p. 1471-7.

[270] Ogden, J. A., E. W. Mee, and M. Henning, A prospective study of impairment of cognition and memory and recovery after subarachnoid hemorrhage. *Neurosurgery,* 1993. 33(4): p. 572-86; discussion 586-7.

[271] Otawara, Y., et al., Comparison of postoperative cognitive function in patients undergoing surgery for ruptured and unruptured intracranial aneurysm. *Surg. Neurol.*, 2009. 72(6): p. 592-5; discussion 595.

[272] Garraway, W. M., J. P. Whisnant, and I. Drury, The changing pattern of survival following stroke. *Stroke,* 1983. 14(5): p. 699-703.

[273] Bonita, R. and S. Thomson, Subarachnoid hemorrhage: epidemiology, diagnosis, management, and outcome. *Stroke,* 1985. 16(4): p. 591-4.

[274] Giroud, M., et al., Incidence and survival rates during a two-year period of intracerebral and subarachnoid hemorrhages, cortical infarcts, lacunes and transient ischaemic attacks. The Stroke Registry of Dijon: 1985-1989. *Int. J. Epidemiol.,* 1991. 20(4): p. 892-9.

[275] Bonita, R., R. Beaglehole, and J. D. North, Subarachnoid hemorrhage in New Zealand: an epidemiological study. *Stroke,* 1983. 14(3): p. 342-7.

[276] Kiyohara, Y., et al., Incidence and prognosis of subarachnoid hemorrhage in a Japanese rural community. *Stroke,* 1989. 20(9): p. 1150-5.

[277] Bamford, J., et al., A prospective study of acute cerebrovascular disease in the community: the Oxfordshire Community Stroke Project--1981-86. 2. Incidence, case fatality rates and overall outcome at one year of cerebral infarction, primary intracerebral and subarachnoid hemorrhage. *J. Neurol. Neurosurg. Psychiatry,* 1990. 53(1): p. 16-22.

[278] Inagawa, T., et al., Study of aneurysmal subarachnoid hemorrhage in Izumo City, Japan. *Stroke,* 1995. 26(5): p. 761-6.

[279] Inagawa, T., et al., Primary intracerebral and aneurysmal subarachnoid hemorrhage in Izumo City, Japan. Part II: management and surgical outcome. *J. Neurosurg.,* 2000. 93(6): p. 967-75.

[280] Truelsen, T., et al., Changes in subarachnoid hemorrhage mortality, incidence, and case fatality in New Zealand between 1981-1983 and 1991-1993. *Stroke,* 1998. 29(11): p. 2298-303.

[281] Anderson, C. S., et al., Predicting survival for 1 year among different subtypes of stroke. Results from the Perth Community Stroke Study. *Stroke*, 1994. 25(10): p. 1935-44.

[282] Kapapa, T. and E. Rickels, Lebensqualität nach spontaner Subarachnoidalblutung. *Neurol. Rehabil.,* 2005. 11(1): p. 21-28.

[283] Katati, M. J., et al., Description of quality of life and its predictors in patients with aneurysmal subarachnoid hemorrhage. *Cerebrovasc. Dis.,* 2007. 24(1): p. 66-73.

[284] Visser-Meily, J. M., et al., Long-term health-related quality of life after aneurysmal subarachnoid hemorrhage: relationship with psychological

symptoms and personality characteristics. *Stroke,* 2009. 40(4): p. 1526-9.

[285] Proust, F., et al., Quality of life and brain damage after microsurgical clip occlusion or endovascular coil embolization for ruptured anterior communicating artery aneurysms: neuropsychological assessment. *J. Neurosurg.,* 2009. 110(1): p. 19-29.

In: Subarachnoid Hemorrhage
Editor: Linda R. Gray

ISBN: 978-1-63463-492-2

Chapter 4

Cerebral and Spinal Subarachnoid Hemorrhage after Lumbar Puncture

Monica del-Rio-Vellosillo[1*]
and Jose Javier Garcia-Medina[2#]
[1]Senior Consultant Anesthetist, Department of Anesthesia, University Hospital Virgen de la Arrixaca, El Palmar, Murcia, Spain
[2]Senior Consultant, Department of Ophthalmology, University Hospital Reina Sofia, Murcia, Spain and Associate Professor, Department of Ophthalmology and Optometry, University School of Medicine, University of Murcia, Murcia, Spain

Abstract

Lumbar puncture (LP) is a safe technique used in anesthetic, diagnostic and therapeutic procedures with very few complications. Post-dural puncture headache (PDPH) is one of the commonest complications. This headache is due to leakage of cerebrospinal fluid (CSF) through

* Email address: monicadelriov@hotmail.com
# Email address: josegarciam@yahoo.com

dural puncture, which causes the caudal displacement of intracranial structures, leading to intracranial hypotension syndrome.

Headache is often postural with a limited time period and responds to conservative treatment. When this headache is long-lasting, it may be due to other causes like subdural hygroma, subdural hematoma, intracerebral hemorrhages (subarachnoid hemorrhage and intraparenchimal hemorrhage). Some may even appear simultaneously in the same patient or can be associated with other hemorrhagic lesions in the spinal cord (spinal epidural hematoma, spinal subdural hematoma and spinal subarachnoid hematoma (SSH)).

Subarachnoid hemorrhage (SAH) after LP is an unusual complication that requires urgent diagnosis and treatment. The physiopathologic mechanisms behind it are still not completely clear and may be multifactorial. Most presumed trigger events are associated with ruptured intracranial aneurysm, hypertensive disease, arteriovenous malformation (AVM), stress peri-anesthesia, cerebral venous thrombosis, or damaged vessels due to decreasing intracranial pressure and tractions of cerebral structures. Indeed knowing the cause of a small number of cases proves impossible.

The incidence of SAH after LP is unknown, and it is an unusual cause of PDPH after LP. Diagnosis is made according to the patient´s clinical situation, together with presence of blood in the subarachnoid space. This fact is established by a computed tomography (CT) scan that can detect most SAHs, and also helps diagnose other underlying lesions, such as intraparenchimal hemorrhage, AVM and aneurysms.

Most SAHs heal spontaneously, but can occasionally lead to death. However, it is a complication that anesthesiologists, neurologists and other specialists should take into account after LP with a severe, longer headache, or when accompanied by neurological symptoms, because early management of such complications can improve patients´ prognosis.

Introduction

LP is a safe technique used for anesthetic, therapeutic and diagnostic procedures. It was introduced in 1891 by Heinrich Quincke from Germany to treat hydrocephalus, and by W. Essex Wynter from England, to reduce brain pressure in tuberculous meningitis [1, 2].

This technique has very few complications as it involves PDPH, one of the commonest complications of LP, with an incidence of 36.5% [3,4]. The use of atraumatic spinal needles with a small diameter is recommended to lower the risk of PDPH [5]. This headache is due to CSF leakage through the hole in the dura. The main mechanism of headache is brain sinking and traction of sensitive brain pain. Engorgement of cerebral veins and venous sinuses can also be involved and, in some situations, perhaps even the dominant mechanism [6]. It is mostly bilateral and oppressive, and the prone position typically improves it. Its duration is often limited and it responds to conservative treatment (resting in bed, medication for pain). Other associated symptoms usually include nausea, vomiting, visual disturbances, interscapular pain, stiff neck, hearing disorders, vertigo and photophobia [7]. When this headache lasts a long time, it may be related to other causes, such as subdural hematoma and hygroma, and intraparenchimal and SAH [8-15]. These brain injuries may appear simultaneously in the same patient or can be associated with other hemorrhagic lesions in the spinal cord; e.g., spinal epidural hematoma, spinal subdural hematoma and SSH [16-23].

Incidence

Cerebral Subarachnoid Hemorrhage

The real incidence of SAH after LP is unknown, and it is a rare, serious cause of PDPH after LP that requires urgent diagnosis and treatment [24].

Knowing the percentage of SAHs occurring after LP is no easy task because we have isolated only published cases and we do not have information about all the cases that have actually incurred in clinical practice.

Subdural hematoma is the commonest cause of intracranial hemorrhage after LP, followed by intraparenchimal hemorrhage and finally SAH [24].

Spinal Subarachnoid Hemorrhage

Incidence of symptomatic SSH, which occurs exclusively as a complication of LP, is difficult to evaluate. Available information seems to indicate that incidence is very low. Indeed only 26 cases have been documented in the literature reviews done several authors to date [25].

As with SAH, it is also difficult to estimate the percentage of spinal hematomas after LP because complications are not always published, and quite often diagnosis and treatment are made by neurosurgeons after LP with no casual relationship stated between spinal hematoma and the LP performed [22]. SSH is not seen in clinical practice since they are more infrequent spinal hematomas, partly due to the dilutive effect of CSF, and spinal hematomas are more frequent than those localized in the epidural spaces [26].

Mechanisms of Production and Associated Factors

Cerebral Subarachnoid Hemorrhage

The mechanisms of emergence of SAH are not clear and may be multifactorial [24]. Most are associated with ruptured intracranial aneurysm (51-80%), followed by hypertensive disease (10-15%) and AVMs (5-10%). Other causes are peri-anesthesia stress, cerebral venous thrombosis or damage to vessels due to reduced intracranial pressure, together with cerebral downward pull after LP. In this last cause, the outer diameter and tip of the needle may relate to the size of the dural lesion and, thus, to the hypotension magnitude of CSF [27]. Lastly, knowing the cause is not possible in a small percentage (5-10%) of cases [28, 29].

In accordance with Monro-Kellie's doctrine [30, 31], one would hypothesize that reduced intracranial pressure and brain descent could result in the dilation of cerebral veins and the distortion of veins walls respectively. Thus both factors may contribute to the tightness and turbulence of blood circulation in cerebral veins, causing thrombosis [32]. Most SAHs are of an aneurysm origin and non traumatic cortical SAHs are infrequent [33]. However, emergence of SAH in patients with isolated cortical venous thrombosis is not unusual [33-35], although the exact mechanism of SAH in patients with isolated cortical venous thrombosis is unknown. When vein thrombosis is limited to one single cortical vein, blood flow may be guided to the collateral venules surrounding the lesion by the direction of flow being reverted. Blood and pressure build up behind, specifically in the subarachnoid segment of the cortical vein, and may produce rupture of blood vessel walls, which could lead to SAH [36]. Furthermore in patients with dural sinus thrombosis, several or most cortical veins are involved, and access of blood flow to other cortical veins collaterally is limited. This could be the reason why SAH appears to have been less associated with dural sinus thrombosis than with isolated cortical venous thrombosis [36].

Spinal Subarachnoid Hemorrhage

At other times, SAH has appeared in the spinal column after LP. The first surgical description of a hematoma in the subarachnoid space was reported by Plotkin et al. in 1966 [37]. The majority of authors think that SSH after LP is caused by the damage that the needle causes in the small blood vessels entering the subarachnoid space with each nerve root [25].

This complication usually occurs more often when puncture has proven difficult; e.g., in patients with hemostasis disorders, or treated with antiplatelets or anticoagulant drugs [37, 38]. Although presence of thrombocytopenia in these patients is considered a risk factor of bleeding after LP, it has not been possible to establish a platelet count limit, which would increase this risk. On occasion, rather than quantitative elements, alterations of hemostasis being caused by functional defects of platelets is hardly objectivable [39, 40]. No evidence-based clinical guidelines are available to recommend guidelines to correct thrombocytopenia before performing LP. Wirtz et al. [40] recommended performing a platelets transfusion if the platelet count was below 50 000 platelets.mm^{-3}, and Edelson et al. [39] recommended this when the platelet count was less than 20 000 platelets.mm^{-3} or when it dropped quickly in subsequent analyses. Traumatic LP may be minimized by using a technique that is as atraumatic as possible and using needles with a minimum diameter [41, 42]. Other risk factors associated with SSH are AVMs and tumors [16].

In this vascular network of the cauda equine, the accidental puncture of the Adamkiewicz vein, this being the main vein usually located around nerve roots L3 and L4, may be the origin of some hematomas, particularly when the needle is guided very laterally [39, 43-45]. Nevertheless, root vessels are often the most likely source of post-LP bleeding [46]. The greater or lesser laceration of the arachnoid would explain the hematoma extending toward the subdural or subarachnoid space, or both at the same time [47].

While SSHs are usually localized, they may also spread in the spinal cord and achieve SAH through migration of blood from the spinal canal to the intracranial space [18-21, 43]. This may be favored by the fact that the blood in the subarachnoid space is mixed with CSF to become more fluid [28].

Blood passing toward cerebral ventricles is extremely unusual. Stügben considered that three conditions were necessary to produce such migration: 1) head displacement of blood; 2) free communication between cistern magna and the IV ventricle; 3) strong resistance in the drainage pathways of CSF in either basal cisterns or brain convexity [48].

Diagnosis

Intracranial Hypotension

The diagnosis is based on the patient´s clinical and medical history, together with typical brain magnetic resonance imaging (MRI).

All the brain MRI findings would result from a pressure drop in CSF. In this way, vascular expansion is valued, which appears to compensate the reduction in CSF [49-51]. This leads to pachymeningeal enhancement and to the expansion of cerebral venous sinuses, which are sometimes accompanied by inferior brain displacement. Brain sagging is associated with diminished ventricle size, effacement of perichiasmatic cisterns with a bowing optic chiasm over the pituitary fossa, effacement of the prepontine cistern with a flattening of pons against the clivus, and downward cerebellar tonsils displacement [11, 52]. Pituitary hyperemia, caused by the expansion of the venous plexus around, may also appear [53], as can subdural fluid collections in a small percentage of cases.

According to Monro-Kellie´s hypothesis, the sum of the volumes of CSF, intracranial blood and cerebral volume must remain constant in a full skull [30, 31]. Therefore in cases with hypovolemia of CSF, a compensatory increase in brain volume at the expense of vascular bed expansion occurs, particularly by veins and venous sinuses [30, 31]. In this way, CSF diminished with no loss of intracranial pressure.

Location and Extension of CSF Leakage

In order to locate the CSF leakage site, we carried out radionuclide cisternography and myelography with an iodinated contrast.

In the radionuclide cisternography, the marking isotopes introduced into CSF included a slow accent along the spinal axis and activity shortage around the brain convexities, so it appears early in the kidney and urinary bladder [54]. In some cases, radionuclide cisternography has allowed the location of CSF leakage. However its use is limited due to its small resolution. The leakage site is unknown in up to one third of patients in whom leakage has been checked by myelography [55].

Nevertheless, myelography with an iodinated contrast, followed by thin slices in CT of all the spinal axes, has proven more sensitive than radionuclide cisternography, and is the study of choice to define exactly the location and extension of CSF leakage [56, 57].

Myelography with intrathecal administration of gadolinium is an excellent alternative [58, 59].

Fear of the brain herniation caused by performing LP through myelography is completely theoretical and has never been documented. The dural hole performed by LP is not only small, but CSF pressure is already low [55].

Cerebral Subarachnoid Hemorrhage

When a patient develops a headache of difficult management after LP, together with other neurological signs and symptoms such as seizures, changes in alertness, meningeal irritation, signs of lateralization, etc., another elementary or side pathology of the central nervous system (CNS) should be suspected, such as brain bleeding. In this situation, it is vital not to delay doing a brain imaging test to obtain an early diagnosis.

Diagnosis is made based on the patient´s clinical situation, together with the demonstration of blood in the subarachnoid space. Clinical SAH symptoms often include occipital headache with sudden, severe and constant onset, unilateral ocular pain, ptosis, weak consciousness, vomiting and stiff neck [60].

A brain CT using a contrast allows the detection of over 95% of SAHs, and also enables the diagnosis of other underlying lesions, such as intraparenchimal hemorrhage, AVMs and aneurysms [24]. An arteriography can be done to rule out an AVM or aneurysm if the brain CT shows no suspicious image [24].

Spinal Subarachnoid Hemorrhage

In SSH, clinical symptoms often include back pain, with or without irradiation by radicular possessions, followed by the appearance of spinal cord or cauda equine compression after a variable period of time (20 minutes-10 days) [16,25]. Sometimes consciousness, meningeal signs and symptoms or seizures can occur [37]. However, these intracranial symptoms may make it difficult to distinguish between an SAH and SSH [37].

Formation of SSH with enough volume to produce a radicular and/or spinal cord compressive syndrome is an extremely rare event in clinical practice. This is explained by many reasons, such as the speed of blood dilution in CSF and its pulsatility, which can prevent blood clots from forming after bleeding. In addition, CSF's own fibrinolytic activity is also enhanced by presence of blood [39, 47, 61].

The clinical signs and neuroradiological characteristics of SSH are often difficult to separate from more common spinal subdural hematoma characteristics. In myelography, the most significant and distinguishable vision is "capping", as illustrated by Frager et al. [62].

MRI is currently the diagnostic imaging test recommended to diagnose SSH. It is well-known that this technique offers greater anatomic detail in spinal pathology and a greater delimitation compared with other tests. The signal characteristics of blood with its different degradation stages in MRI offers high sensitivity and specificity while diagnosing bleeding [43,63,64]. Despite the cause-and-effect relationship being clear in post-LP hematoma cases, it is advisable to perform MRI sequences with an intravenous contrast to rule out any underlying injuries.

MRI well defines the extension of an SSH after LP, and it usually covers several vertebral levels of lower back and dorsal areas, which affect the conus medullaris and cauda equine [25]. However, despite all the advantages that this test offers, in many cases neither this nor other radiological examinations can distinguish if a spinal intradural hematoma is localized in the subdural space, the subarachnoid space, or even in both [65]. This precision may be of interest for planning and for the results to study possible surgical treatment.

Treatment and Prognosis

Post Dural Puncture Headache

The main complication of LP is PDPH. In some cases however, there may be associated complications that threaten life, such as uncal herniation and uncontrollable bleeding confined to the CNS [66].

Regarding PDPH, its initial treatment is symptomatic: rest in bed, abundant hydration, caffeine, analgesics and steroidal drugs. However, if a postural headache persists or is disabling, especially if other neurological symptoms are associated, epidural treatments (autologous blood, physiological saline, dextranes, fibrin, etc.) are the right choice.

The mechanism of action of an epidural blood patch is divided into immediate effect (increase of volume with elevated CSF pressure) and late effect (formation of an organized blood clot to repair the dural defect and to prevent CSF leakage) [67]. The right amount of blood to perform an epidural blood patch varies from 10 to 15 ml. This volume can spread from 8 to 10 segments from the site of its placement (six segments in the cephalic direction and three caudally), with a medium magnitude of one spinal segment per 1.6 ml of blood [67]. Injection is done at a speed of 1 ml.3 sec^{-1} and it must finish when the patient reports discomfort at the back or legs before reaching 15 ml. This pain is due to the traction or irritation of a nerve root by the blood clot, which may last 2-5 days [67]. Other options include the intermittent epidural infusion of 0.9% physiological saline (bolus of 30-50 ml) or continuous infusion (25-30 $ml.h^{-1}$). Nevertheless it can be transient and insufficient to correct the inherent defect, and it is sometimes necessary to perform other treatments to achieve eventual relief of symptoms [68]. Epidural dextrans (20-30 mg of dextran 40) have proven that 64% of PDPHs do not recur [69]. An epidural patch with the fibrin adhesive system has achieved promising results and could be a good alternative [70].

Overall, the response to the epidural blood patch is immediate in at least 30% of cases [24]. If the first epidural blood patch fails, a second epidural blood patch is performed after at least 5 days have elapsed since the first epidural blood patch was done [24]. If at all possible, the CSF leakage site will be localized with a cisternogram or a myelogram, which is performed as closely as possible to the injury [67]. Finally, surgery should be used only in those cases in which many epidural patches have failed and when the location of the CSF fistula has been radiologically verified [71].

Cerebral Subarachnoid Hemorrhage

Despite an SAH after LP being an infrequent complication, it is serious. It resolves on its own, but may have devastating results, and can even lead to the patient´s death, as noted in some published case reports as a complication of LP [10, 17, 48].

Such cerebral hemorrhaging can cause severe brain dysfunction as a result of increased intracranial pressure, encephalitis, aseptic meningitis, cerebral vasospasm or mass effect [72-76], and surgery is the treatment considered in such cases. In other published cases, SAH size was small and the patient did not require surgery [11]. Thus the clinical management of these patients must be personalized.

Spinal Subarachnoid Hemorrhage

Treatment of SSH depends on the patient's clinical and neurological circumstances. If the neurologic deficit is significant or progressive, and the clinical situation allows it, the treatment of choice consists in decompressive laminectomy and in evacuating the hematoma as soon as possible as the time before it is done is closely related with the recovery opportunities of the neurological deficit [16, 77].

Minimally invasive techniques have been proposed as an alternative to laminectomy with satisfactory outcomes. In this way, Schwerdtfeger et al. [78], was able to not only evacuate an SSH by inserting an intrathecal catheter, but to also produce irrigations and repeated suctions. In patients with minor neurological affectation, it is possible to adopt a wait-and-see approach, together with clinical radiological follow-up [79]. In these cases, spontaneous resolutions of hematomas with excellent functional results have been verified [25].

The factors with worse reported neurological prognosis include delayed surgical treatment and presence of a full compressive syndrome (abolition of sensitive, motor and sphincter functions) [25].

Some authors have suggested that ventral SSH localization is a good prognosis factor [80], but this has not been corroborated by others [64]. Finally, Domenicucci et al. [81] observed in their study that intradural hematomas with a subarachnoid component obtained a worse prognosis than those with no subarachnoid component.

SAH and SSH are two complications that should be considered by anesthesiologists, neurologists and other specialists after LP since the early management of these complications can improve patients' prognoses.

References

[1] Quincke H. *Die Lumbal punction Des Hydrocephalus*. Berlin: August Hirschwald; 1891.

[2] Wynter W. Four cases of tubercular meningitis in which paracentesis of the theca vertebralis was performed for the relief of fluid pressure. *Lancet*. 1891;1:981-2.

[3] Benzon HT, Wong CA. Postdural puncture headache: mechanisms, treatment, and prevention. *Reg Anesth Pain Med*. 2001;26:293-5.

[4] Kuntz KM, Kokmen E, Stevens JC, Miller P, Offord KP, Ho MM. Post-LP headaches: experience in 501 consecutive procedures. *Neurology*. 1992;42:1884-7.

[5] Armon C, Evans RW. Prevention of post-lumbar puncture headaches: report of the Therapeutics and Technology Assessment Subcommittee of the American Academy of Neurology. *Neurology*. 2005;65:510-2.

[6] Mokri B. Spontaneous low pressure, low CSF volume headaches: spontaneous CSF leaks. *Headache*. 2013;53:1034-53.

[7] Bleeker CP, Hendriks IM, Booij LH. Postpartum post-dural puncture headache: is your differential diagnosis complete? *Br J Anaesth*. 2004;93:461-4.

[8] Jonsson LO, Einarsson P, Olsson GL. Subdural haematoma and spinal anaesthesia: a case report and an incidence study. *Anaesthesia*. 1983;38:144-6.

[9] Vos PE, de Boer WA, Wurzer JA, van Gijn J. Subdural haematoma after lumbar puncture: two case reports and review of the literatura. *Clin Neurol Neurosurg*. 1991; 93:127-32.

[10] Acharya R, Chhabra SS, Ratra M, Sehgal AD. Cranial subdural haematoma after spinal anaesthesia. *Br J Anaesth*. 2001;86:893-5.

[11] Del-Rio-Vellosillo M, Garcia-Medina JJ, Fernandez-Rodriguez LE, Martin-Gil-Parra R, Lopez-Perez J, Almagro-Navarro MJ. Subdural hygroma accompanied by parenchymal and subarachnoid hemorrhage after epidural analgesia in an obstetric patient. *Acta Anaesthesiol Scand*. 2014;58:897-902.

[12] Van den Berg JS, Sijbrandy SE, Meijer AH, Oostdijk AH. Subdural hygroma: a rare complication of spinal anesthesia. *Anesth Analg*. 2002;94:1625-7.

[13] Verdu M, Alonso B, Burguillos S, Martinez-Lage JF. Postpartum subdural hygroma after epidural analgesia. *Anesthesiology*. 1999;91: 867-9.

[14] Openshaw H, Ressler JA, Snyder DS. Lumbar puncture and subdural hygroma and hematomas in hematopoietic cell transplant patients. *Bone Marrow Transplantation*. 2008;41:791-5.

[15] Aragones N, Arxer A, Vieito M, Ros J, Villalonga A, Ustrell X. The diagnosis and treatment of a patient with puerperal infection and subdural hygromas. *Anesth Analg*. 2004; 99:1218-20.

[16] Peiro CM, Caballer N, Errando CL, Moliner S. Hematoma espinal y cerebral postpunción lumbar diagnóstica con evolución letal. *Rev Esp Anestesiol Reanim*. 2003; 50: 481-5.

[17] Walsh MN, Fischer GG, Anderson D, Mastri A. Fatal intracranial extension of spinal hemorrhage after lumbar puncture. *Arch Neurol*. 1984;41:987-9.

[18] Liu WH, Lin JH, Lin JC, Ma HI. Severe intracranial and intraspinal subarachnoid hemorrhage after lumbar puncture: a rare case report. *Am J Emerg Med*. 2008 ;26:633.e1-3

[19] Hans GA, Senard M, Ledoux D, Grayet B, Scholtes F, Creemers E, Lamy ML. Cerebral subarachnoid blood migration consecutive to a lumbar haematoma after spinal anaesthesia. *Acta Anaesthesiol Scand*. 2008;52:1021-3.

[20] Rocchi R, Lombardi C, Marradi I, Di Paolo M, Cerase A. Intracranial and intraspinal hemorrhage following spinal anesthesia. *Neurol Sci*. 2009;30:393-6.

[21] Espinosa-Aguilar M, Hernández-Palazón J, Fuentes-García D. Intraspinal and intracranial subarachnoid hemorrhage with severe cerebral vasospasm after spinal anaesthesia for assisted delivery. *Br J Anaesth*. 2012;108:885-6.

[22] Lee SJ, Lin YY, Hsu CW, Chu SJ, Tsai SH. Intraventricular hematoma, subarachnoid hematoma and spinal epidural hematoma caused by lumbar puncture: an unusual complication. *Am J Med Sci*. 2009;337:143-5.

[23] Lee AC, Lau Y, Li CH, Wong YC, Chiang AK. Intraspinal and intracranial hemorrhage after lumbar puncture. *Pediatr Blood Cancer*. 2007;48:233-7.

[24] Prats-Vinas JM, Garcia-Ribes A, Suinaga-Errasti I. Spontaneous intracranial hypotension as the cause of persistent headache in a paediatric case. *Rev Neurol*. 2011;53:317-8.

[25] Ayerbe J, Quiñones D, Prieto E, Sousa P. Spinal subarachnoid hematoma after lumbar puncture in a patient with leukemia: report of a case and review of the literature *Neurocirugia*. 2005;16:447-52.

[26] Rengachary SS, Murphy D. Subarachnoid hematoma following lumbar puncture causing compression of the cauda equina. Case report. *J Neurosurg*. 1974;41:252-4.

[27] Reina MA, Lopez A, Benito-León J, Pulido P, María F. Intracranial and spinal subdural hematoma: a rare complication of epidural and subarachnoid anesthesia. *Rev Esp Anestesiol Reanim.* 2004;51:28-39.

[28] De la Linde C. Complicaciones de la anestesia espinal. *Act Anest Reanim (Madrid).* 1997;7:15-26.

[29] Eggert SM, Eggers KA. Subarachnoid hemorrhage following spinal anaesthesia in an obstetric patient. *Br J Anaesth.* 2001;86:442-4.

[30] Bruca OC, Bonamico L, Giglio JA, Sinay V, Leston JA, Figuerola ML. Intracranial Hypotension: The Nonspecific Nature Of MRI Findings. *Headache.* 2000;40:848-52.

[31] Bahram Mokri MD. The Monro-Kellie hypothesis. *Neurology.* 2002;56:1746-8.

[32] Lai PH, Li JY, Lo YK, Wu MT, Liang HL, Chen CK. A case of spontaneous intracranial hypotension complicated by isolated cortical vein thrombosis and cerebral venous infarction. *Cephalalgia.* 2007;27:87-90.

[33] Chang R, Friedman DP. Isolated cortical venous thrombosis presenting as subarachnoid hemorrhage: a report of three cases. *AJNR Am J Neuroradiol.* 2004;25:1676-9.

[34] Urban PP, Müller-Forell W. Clinical and neuroradiological spectrum of isolated cortical vein thrombosis. *J Neurol.* 2005;252:1476-81.

[35] Spitzer C, Mull M, Rohde V, Kosinski CM. Non-traumatic cortical subarachnoid hemorrhage: diagnostic work-up and aetiological background. *Neuroradiology.* 2005;47:525-31.

[36] Wang YF, Fuh JL, Lirng JF, Chang FC, Wang SJ. Spontaneous intracranial hypotension with isolated cortical vein thrombosis and subarachnoid hemorrhage. *Cephalalgia.* 2007;27:1413-7.

[37] Plotkin HB, Ronthal M, Froman C. Spontaneous spinal subarachnoid hemorrhage: report of 3 cases. *J Neurosurg.* 1966;25:443-6.

[38] Paal P, Putz G, Gruber E, Le GT, Lemberger P. Subarachnoid hemorrhage after lumbar puncture in a patient receiving aspirin and clopidrogel. *Anesth Analg.* 2006;102:644-5.

[39] Edelson, R.N., Chernik, N.L., Posner, J.B. Spinal subdural hematoma complicating lumbar puncture: ocurrence in thrombocytopenic patients. *Arch Neurol.* 1974;31:134-7.

[40] Wirtz, P.W., Bloem, B.R., van der Meer, F.J.M., Brouwer, O.F. Paraparesis after lumbar puncture in a male with leukemia. *Pediatr Neurol.* 2000;23:67-8.

[41] Gutterman P. Acute spinal subdural hematoma following lumbar puncture. *Surg Neurol.* 1977;7:355-6.
[42] Reynolds F. Dural puncture and headache. Avoid the first but treat the second. *Br Med J.* 1993;306:874-6.
[43] Kreppel D, Antoniadis G, Seeling W. Spinal hematoma: a literature survey with meta-analysis of 613 patients. *Neurosurg Rev.* 2003;26: 1-49.
[44] Yoshioka K, Niinuma H, Ehara S, Nakajima T, Nakamura M, Kawazoe K. MR angiography and CT angiography of the artery of Adamkiewicz: state of the art. *Radiographic.* 2006;26:S63-73.
[45] Masdeu JC, Breuer AC, Schoene WC. Spinal subarachnoid hematomas: clue to a source of bleeding in traumatic lumbar puncture. *Neurology.* 1979;29:872-6.
[46] Tubbs RS, Smyth MD, Wellons JC 3rd, Oakes WJ. Intramedullary hemorrhage in a neonate after lumbar puncture resulting in paraplegia: a case report. *Pediatrics.* 2004;113:1403-5.
[47] Scott EW, Cazenave CR, Virapongse C. Spinal subarachnoid hematoma complicating lumbar puncture: diagnosis and management. *Neurosurgery.* 1989;25: 287-93.
[48] Stügben JP. Intraventricular blood after "traumatic" lumbar puncture: a report of two cases. *Child's Nerv Syst.* 1995;11:492-3.
[49] 49.Weitz S, Drasner K. Spontaneous intracranial hypotension: A series. *Anesthesiology.* 1996;85:923-5.
[50] Spelle L, Boulin A, Tainturier C, Visot A, Graveleau P, Pierot L. Neuroimaging features of spontaneous intracranial hypotension. *Neuroradiology.* 2001;43:622-7.
[51] Mokri Md. Cerebrospinal fluid volume depletion and its emerging clinical/imaging syndromes. *Neurosurg Focus.* Vol. 9. July, 2000.
[52] Pannullo SC, Reich JB, Krol G, Deck MDF, Posner JB. MRI changes in intracranial hypotension. *Neurology.* 1993;43:919-26.
[53] Alvarez-Linera J, Escribano J, Benito-leon J, Porta-Etessam J, Rovira A. Pituitary enlargement in patients with intracranial hypotension síndrome. *Neurology.* 2000;55: 1895-7.
[54] Jeon TJ, Lee JD, Lee BI, Kim DI, Yoo HS. Radionuclide cisternography in spontaneous intracranial hypotension with simultaneous leaks at the cervocothoracic and lumbar levels. *Clin Nucl Med.* 2001;26:1083-128.
[55] Schievink WI. Spontaneous spinal cerebrospinal fluid leaks. *Cephalalgia.* 2008;28:1345-56.

[56] Morki B, Piepgras D, Miller G. Syndrome of orthostatic headache and diffuse pachymeningeal gadolinium enhancement. *Mayo Clin Proc.* 1997;72:400-13.

[57] Schievink WI, Meyer FB, Atkinson JL, Mokri B. Spontaneous spinal cerebrospinal fluid leaks and intracranial hypotension. *J Neurosurg.* 1996;84:598-605.

[58] Liong WC, Constantinescu CS, Jaspan T. Intrathecal gadolinium-enhanced magnetic resonance myelography in the detection of CSF leak. *Neurology.* 2006;67:1522.

[59] Albayram S, Kilic F, Ozer H, Baghaki S, Kocer N, Islak C. Gadolinium-enhanced MR cisternography to evaluate dural leaks in intracranial hypotension syndrome. *AJNR Am J Neuroradiol.* 2008;29:116-21.

[60] Schoenen J, Maartens de Noordhout A. Headache. In: Wall PD, Melzack R, eds. Textbook of Pain. New York, NY: Churchill Living-stone, 1985; 495-521.

[61] Blade J, Gaston F, Montserrat E, Marin P, Grañena A, Bachs A, Rozman C. Spinal subarachnoid hematoma after lumbar puncture causing reversible paraplegia in acute leukemia. Case report. *J Neurosurg.* 1983;58:438-9.

[62] Frager D, Zimmerman RD, Wisoff HS, Leeds NE. Spinal subarachnoid hematoma. *AJNR Am J Neuroradiol.* 1982;3:77-9.

[63] Kulkarni AV, Willinsky RA, Gray T, Cusimano M. Serial magnetic resonance imaging findings for a spontaneously resolving spinal subdural hematoma: case report. *Neurosurgery.* 1998;42:398-400.

[64] Ruelle A, Zerbi D, Andrioli G. Spinal subarachnoid bleeding of unknown etiology. Case repots. *J Neurosurg Sci.* 2001;45:53-7.

[65] Hausmann O, Kirsch E, Radü E, Mindermann Th, Gratzl O. Coagulopathy induced spinal intradural extramedullary haematoma: report of three cases and review of the literature. *Acta Neurochir.* 2001;143:135-40.

[66] Ellenby MS, Tegtmeyer K, Lai S, Braner DA. Lumbar puncture. *N Engl J Med.* 2006;335:e12.

[67] Lopez-Sanchez F, Asensio I, Molina I, Barrio J, Sanchez-Roy R, Garcia-Ferrando V. Parche sanguíneo epidural como tratamiento de un cuadro de hipotension intracranial espontanea. *Rev. Soc. Esp. Dolor.* 2003;10:511-5.

[68] Arjona A. Prevention and treatment of headache due to intracranial hypotension. *Rev Neurol.* 1998; 27:1027-33.

[69] Silberstein SD. Headache associated with low cerebrospinal fluid pressure. Thomas Jefferson University Hospital. Philadelphia, PA. Kamada M, Fujita Y, Ishii R, Endoh S. Spontaneous intracranial hypotension successfully treated by epidural patching with fibrin glue. *Headache*. 2000;40:844-7.

[70] Maher C, Meyer F, Mokri B. Surgical treatment of spontaneous spinal cerebrospinal fluid leaks. Neurosurg. Focus/Volume 9/July, 2000.

[71] Satoskar AR, Goel A, Desai AP, Usgaonkar TA. Intracranial haemorrhage and death after iohexol myelography. *J Neurol Neurosurg Psychiatry*. 1991;54:1118-20.

[72] May A, Faiss J, KeidelM, Schwarz M, Weiller C. Severe neurological complications following lumbar myelography. *Nervenarzt*. 1994;65:125-7.

[73] Smith RA, Collier HF, Underwood FO. Cerebral vasospasm following myelography. *Surg Neurol*. 1973;1:87-90.

[74] Ceylan S, Baykal S, Kuzeyli K, Akturk F, Komsuoglu S. A case of acute encephalopathy after iohexol lumbar myelography. *Clin Neurol Neurosurg*. 1993;95:45-7.

[75] DonaghyM, Fletcher NA, Schott GD. Encephalopathy after iohexol myelography. *Lancet*. 1985;2:887.

[76] Domenicucci M, Ramieri A, Ciappetta P, Delfini R. Nontraumatic acute spinal subdural hematoma: report of five cases and review of the literature. *J Neurosurg*. 1999;91:65-73.

[77] Schwerdtfeger K, Caspar W, Alloussi S, Strowitzki M, Loew F. Acute spinal intradural extramedullary hematoma: a nonsurgical approach for spinal cord decompression. *Neurosurgery*. 1990;27:312-4.

[78] Groen RJM. Non-operative treatment of spontaneous spinal epidural hematomas: A review of the literature and a comparison with operative cases. *Acta Neurochir*. 2004;146:103-10.

[79] Komiyama M, Yasui T, Sumimoto T, Fu, Y. Spontaneous spinal subarachnoid hematoma of unknown pathogenesis: case reports. *Neurosurgery*. 1997;41:691-4.

[80] Domenicucci M, Ramieri A, Paolini S, Russo N, Occhiogrosso G, Di Biasi C, Delfini R. Spinal subarachnoid hematomas: our experience and literature review. *Acta Neurochir (Wien)*. 2005;147:741–50.

In: Subarachnoid Hemorrhage
Editor: Linda R. Gray
ISBN: 978-1-63463-492-2

Chapter 5

Long-Term Health Outcomes of Subarachnoid Hemorrhage

Suzanne Barker-Collo[1], Rita Krishnamurthi[2], Flora Minsun Suh[3] and Valery Feigin[2]
[1]School of Psychology,The University of Auckland, Auckland, New Zealand
[2]National Institute of Stroke and Applied Neurorehabilitation (NISAN), AUT University, Auckland, New Zealand
[3]Department of Psychology, The University of Queensland, Australia

Abstract

Subarachnoid Hemorrhage (SAH) constitutes approximately 5% of all strokes (Longstreth, Koepsell, Yerby & van Belle, 1985) and affects 21,000-33,000 people every year in the United States (Rosamond et al., 2007). Though constituting only a small proportion of incident stroke cases, SAH has a higher case fatality than other stroke types with 28-day case fatality reported as 12% for ischemic stroke, 45% for intracerebral haemorrhage, 50% for SAH and 38% for stroke of undermined type (Thrift et al., 2001). In the absence of appropriate interventions, the number of deaths due to stroke worldwide is expected to rise to 6.5 million in 2015 and to 7.8 million in 2030 (Strong, Mathers & Bonita, 2007). As SAH outcomes tend to change overtime (Haug et al., 2007; Koivisto et al., 2000), studying SAH over time is important from the stand-point of better understanding its natural course and the impact of various management strategies. Studying long-term outcomes of SAH in a population based context is important, yet there are few population based studies of SAH survivors beyond 12 months (Hackett & Anderson, 2000) and even fewer examining wider outcomes such as neuropsychological outcomes, quality of life (Mocco et al., 2006), disability (Hop, Rinkel, Algra & van Gijn, 1997), and mood (Powell, Kitchen, Heslin & Greenwood, 2004). This chapter will review the existing literature on long-term (> 12 months) health outcomes of SAH with a focus on these less evidenced outcomes; including neuropsychological functioning, quality of life, and disability; placing these within the context of the WHO models of health.

Model of Health Outcomes

In health outcomes research, outcomes are measured from different perspectives, and a number of models of human functioning and disability have been applied (Albrecht, Sleeman & Bury, 2001; Jette, 2006). The most commonly used framework of outcomes is the International Classification of Impairments, Disabilities and Handicaps (ICIDH; World Health Organization [WHO], 1980) and its' replacement the International Classification of Functioning, Disability and Health (ICF; WHO, 2001)

The WHO recognised that the existing medical model and the International Classification of Diseases (ICD) was useful for classifying medical diagnosis, but inadequate to address disability as it neglected the consequences of disease (Fougeyrollas, 1995). With no consensus on the understanding of health outcomes, the WHO developed the International Classification of Impairments, Disabilities, and Handicaps (ICIDH) for use in conjunction with the ICD (WHO, 1980). The main aim of the ICIDH was to present a model of cause and effect relationships between levels of impact or conceptual levels. According to this model, injury/disease leads to functional and organic impairment and is associated with signs and symptoms, "In the context of health experience, an *impairment* is any loss or abnormality of psychological, physiological, or anatomical structure or function" (WHO, 1980, p.27). These impairments results in disability in an individual's behaviour and activities, where "a *disability* is any restriction or lack (resulting from an impairment) of ability to perform an activity in the manner or within the range considered normal for a human being" (WHO, 1980, p. 28); such as the inability to dress independently. Finally, "a *handicap* is a disadvantage for a given individual, resulting from an impairment or a disability, that limits or prevents the fulfilment of a role that is normal (based on age, sex, and social and cultural factors) for that individual" (WHO, 1980, p. 29); such as job loss or marital breakdown arising as a consequence of disease.

Although the ICIDH is an important and widely used framework for classifying function and disability associated with health conditions (Badley, 1993), it failed to receive endorsement from the World Health Assembly (Stucki, 2005). The major criticism was the linearity of the model as it progressed from biomedical to psychosocial constructs (i.e., from impairments to disabilities to handicaps); failing to clarify the causal and temporal relationship between the three dimensions (Gray & Hendershot, 2000; Johnston & Pollard, 2001). Furthermore, the three 'levels' overlap (Badley, 1993), and insufficient attention is given to the role of the environment in an individual's outcome (Fougeyrollas, 1995). For example, an individual unable to walk might be able to mobilize using a wheelchair; but could not do so in settings without wheelchair access or obstacles to wheelchair use.

To address these criticisms, the WHO developed a revised classification, the International Classification of Functioning, Disability and Health (ICF; see figure 1). The ICF provides a framework and standard language for classifying and describing health and health related states, both at individual and population levels (Jette, 2006; Stucki, 2005) and was endorsed by the 54th World Health Assembly (WHO, 2001). In this model '*Body functions*' are physiological and psychological functions of the body systems (e.g., memory), while anatomical parts of the body are '*body structures*' (e.g., brain structures, limbs). Abnormality in body functions or structures is referred to as 'impairment'. '*Activity'* is the execution of a task by the individual, including their capacity and actual performance of the task. Difficulties executing activities is referred as 'activity limitation' (e.g., difficulty walking due to mobility limitations). Finally, *'participation'* refers to involvement in life situations. Problems experienced by an individual with such involvements are called 'participation restriction' (e.g., restricted social life due to walking difficulty). *Environmental* factors include physical, social and attitudinal factors such as products, technology, supports, relationships, attitudes, available services, social systems and policies which can facilitate or hinder a person's level of function and disability. *Personal factors* include the individual's background and do not include their health condition (e.g., age, sex, ethnicity, coping style).

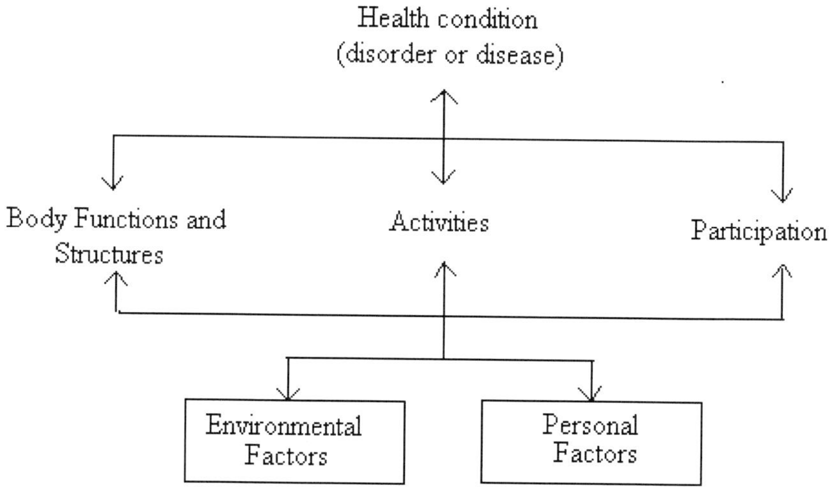

Figure 1. The current framework of Functioning, Disability and Health (ICF).

Thus, the focus of the ICF is on activities of an individual, their participation and contribution to the social environment. The ICF framework is comprehensive, with universally accepted terminology for functioning and disability (Stucki, 2005) and has been implemented in many countries in various sectors (Cieza et al., 2006; Jette, 2006; Stucki, Cieza & Melvin, 2007; WHO, 2001). One of the main criticisms of the ICF is that it cannot be consistently applied to clinical practice as it contains over 1400 categories (Üstün, Chatterji & Kostanjsek, 2004). To improve clinical applicability, ICF Core Sets were developed "to select sets of categories out of the whole classification, which can serve as minimal standards of assessment, communication and reporting of functioning and health for clinical studies, clinical encounters and multi-professional comprehensive assessment and management purposes" (Grill, Ewert, Chatterji, Kostanjsek & Stucki 2005, p 362). A comprehensive ICF Core Set for stroke has been developed, which includes 41 body functions, 5 body structures, 51 activities and participation, and 33 environment factors (Geyh et al., 2004). However, this core set needs to be validated. Thus far, inter-rater reliability of the ICF core sets for stroke has been found to be moderate (Starrost et al., 2008). A recent study suggests the ICF stroke core set be reduced to 28 body functions, and 41 activities and participation components to enhance feasibility for assessment (Algurén, Lundgren-Nilsson & Sunnerhagen, 2010). Another recent study has supported the construct validity of the 'functioning' part of the ICF stroke core set (Ewert, Allen, Wislon, Üstün & Stucki, 2010).

In this chapter, we explore the long-term outcomes (>12 months) of SAH across the three primary ICF categories of body functioning (measures of impairment: neuropsychological tests and mood), activity (measures of disability), and participation (health related quality of life [HRQoL]). In the ensuing section outcomes of SAH are reviewed within the ICF framework and the following labels are used: impairment (body functioning), disability (activity) and handicap (participation) to avoid confusion and for consistency.

SAH Outcomes

As SAH outcomes tend to change overtime (Haug et al., 2007; Koivisto et al., 2000), studying long-term outcomes of SAH is important from the stand-point of better understanding its natural course and impact of various preventative and management interventions. Studying long-term outcomes of SAH in a population based context is important, yet there are few population based studies of SAH survivors beyond 12 months (Hackett & Anderson, 2000); and even fewer examining wider outcomes such as neuropsychological outcomes, quality of life (Mocco et al., 2006), disability (Hop, Rinkel, Algra & van Gijn, 1997), and mood (Powell, Kitchen, Heslin & Greenwood, 2004). The following section reviews these areas of long-term outcomes of SAH. Greater attention is given to cognitive and functional outcomes and to population based studies where these are available.

Cognitive Outcomes

Neuropsychological functioning may be defined as the way in which brain functioning is reflected in behaviour (Lezak, Howieson & Loring, 2004) including planning, memory, information processing speed, and language abilities. Neuropsychological impairments are an important sequel of stroke, occurring in 30-65% of the stroke survivors (Ballard, Rowan, Stephens, Kalaria & Kenney, 2003; Srikanth et al., 2003). Previous research indicates that although 70-80% of the SAH patients survive surgery with positive neurological outcome (Uski et al., 2000), approximately 60% have considerable cognitive impairment (Hütter, Gilsbach & Kreitschmann-Andermahr, 1995; Saciri & Kos, 2002).

Cognitive impairment has been reported in up to 83% of SAH survivors (Mavaddat, Sahakian, Hutchinson & Kirkpatrick, 1999). Despite good neurological outcome, persistent cognitive consequences may manifest years after SAH (Mavaddat et al., 1999), impacting participation and psychosocial functioning (Ravnik et al., 2006). While SAH survivors tend to experience ongoing problems, recovery of cognitive function is a process with different time courses for different areas of impairment (Haug et al. 2007; Koivisto et al. 2000; Ogden, Mee & Henning, 1993). For example, Frazer, Ahuja, Watkins and Cipolotti (2007) examined the cognitive outcome of SAH survivors during the post-acute stage and at 6-months follow-up, reporting significant improvements in intellectual functioning, memory, executive functions, and speed of processing. Recovery is impacted by environmental and personal factors, and may involve developing appropriate coping skills, and is influenced by having a positive attitude towards recovery (Ogden, Utley & Mee, 1997).

Similarly, Koivisto et al., (2000) report that cognitive performance of SAH patients improved across assessments conducted 3 months and 12 months post-SAH (Koivisto et al., 2000). Studies have reported that cognitive recovery continues beyond 3-months; with a plateau starting at 9-months and lasting until 15-months (Samra et al., 2007). However, cognitive deficits are still present up to 5-years post-SAH (Cheng, Shi & Zhou, 2006). Unfortunately, as compared to the acute phase of SAH, very little data is available on long-term cognitive consequences as most studies are limited to short-term (≤6-months) follow-up (Mayer et al., 2002; Uski et al., 2000), participants are referred to hospital and/or rehabilitation settings introducing selection bias, and given its relatively low incidence some studies have small sample sizes (e.g., N=16; Ogden, Levin & Mee, 1990).

Since SAH outcomes are thought to change over time, studying SAH longitudinally is important for better understanding its natural course, the changing needs of survivors, and its impact on family and society. For this, a detailed neuropsychological assessment is extremely valuable. Table 1 presents a summary of studies which have examined long-term (> 12 months) cognitive outcomes of SAH focusing on studies that used a neuropsychological battery rather than single brief screening measures such as MMSE.

As can be seen in table 1, most of the existing long-term studies on SAH exclude the very old (e.g., Huag et al., 2009; Hütter et al., 1995) and those with severe grades of SAH (e.g., Ravnik et al., 2006). There is evidence that cognitive outcomes in SAH survivors may vary due to injury characteristics such as impact of bleed, SAH severity, recurrent SAH and demographic variables such as age, race, ethnicity, and education (Egge et al., 2004; Haug et al., 2007; Ogden et al., 1993; Scharbrodt, Stein, Schreiber, Böker & Oertel, 2009). For example, mild to moderate cognitive impairment is associated with younger and more educated patients who are most likely to be functioning at higher level before the SAH (Haug et al., 2010; Powell, et al., 2004).

It is also apparent that SAH survivors who make a good clinical recovery or do well on global outcome measures (e.g., Glasgow Outcome Scale score) still exhibit cognitive deficits (Hadjivassiliou et al., 2001; Ogden et al., 1990; Powell et al., 2004; Ravnik et al., 2006). Yet the presence and patterns of cognitive impairments post-SAH vary across studies. Some investigators have found that individuals experience little or no persisting significant neuropsychological deficits after uncomplicated SAH (Germanò et al., 1998; Haug et al., 2009), while others report significant impairment across cognitive domains (Alfieri et al., 2008; Hadjivassiliou et al., 2001; Haug et al., 2010; Ogden et al., 1990). The reasons for these inconsistencies are likely related to variability in samples - studies showing little or no cognitive deficits tend to exclude participants with unfavourable neurological outcome, older age (≥70 years), or presence of aphasia (Germanò et al., 1998; Haug et al., 2009). Memory (verbal and non-verbal) is the most commonly examined domain, perhaps because of its impact on everyday life; and the studies have reported that it is the most frequently impaired cognitive domain post-SAH (Haug et al., 2009; Ravnik et al., 2006; Madureira, Canhão, Guerreiro & Ferro, 2000; Wong et al., 2009).

Mood and Emotion

Having reviewed cognitive outcomes following SAH, this section turns its focus to mood outcomes. Emotional problems are a common consequence of stroke that impact other outcomes and the recovery process (Goodwin & Devanand, 2008; Haacke et al., 2006; Hedlund, Zetterling, Ronne-Engstrom, Ekselius & Carlsson 2010; Kauhanen et al., 1999; Sturm et al., 2004; Townend et al., 2007). Post-stroke depression (PSD) and anxiety (PSA) have received the most attention (Barker-Collo, 2007; Berg, Palomäki, Lehtihalmes, Lönnqvist & Kaste, 2003; Whyte, Mulsant, Vanderbilt, Dodge & Ganguli, 2004; Wilkinson et al., 1997) and have been reported to be present for years after the acute phase (Chausson et al., 2010; Ogden et al., 1990). Although PSA will be reviewed the literature remains scarce, the main focus here will therefore be on PSD.

Table 1. Neuropsychological outcomes using a battery of tests > 12 months post-SAH

Author/study	Sample	Time post-SAH	Measures	Outcome
Haug et al. (2009) *Prospective study*	N=46 Aneurysmal SAH (ACoA, MCA only) $\bar{x}$ Age =53 yrs	1-yr	CVLT-II, CVMT, Grooved Pegboard, WAIS-III (DS, DSy), WASI-R (Vocabulary, Similarities, BD, Matrices), D-KEFS (verbal & design fluency, colour word interference, TMT, sorting)	mild to moderate↓ memory, attention, motor/psycho-motor, intellectual, executive functioning Better functioning in MCA sample
Egge et al. (2005) *Prospective study*	N=42 SAH $\bar{x}$= 28-69 yrs	1-yr	HRTB (SRT, TMT-A/B), WMS-R (verbal and visual paired associates), COWAT, WCST (computerised), Grooved Pegboard	normal cognition 7% 93% ↓ memory, information processing, cognitive flexibility, problem solving
Ogden et al. (1990) *Prospective study*	N= 16 SAH $\bar{x}$ =50 yrs	5-yrs	NART, WAIS-R (Vocabulary, comprehension, BD, DS, DSy), WMS (LM, VR, PA), RCFT, WCST (modified), TT, visuospatial neglect tests, MTDDA, EHT	Cognition ↓ (mild-severe): memory, visuospatial, executive functioning 37.5% ↓ in < 2 domains 25% ↓ in 3-4 domains 37.5% ↓ in > 5 domains
Hütter and Gilsbach (1993) *Retrospective study*	N= 31 Aneurysmal SAH $\bar{x}$=42.9 yrs	$\bar{x}$=3-yrs	WIF, d2 (concentration), LPS-LD, LPS-RV, IST, BT, FWIT, TT, WD, HWIE	-Cognitive ↓ 7%-62% -54% ↓ in >3 domains -25% ↓ in 5-7 domains Most ↓ attention, then memory No ↓ general intelligence
Hütter et al. (1995) *Retrospective study*	N=58 SAH $\bar{x}$= 46 yrs	3-yrs	WIF, d2 (concentration), LPS-LD, LPS-RV, IST, BT, FWIT, TT, WD, HWIE	42% cognitively ↓ Maximum ↓: visual short term memory (46%), attention (65%), verbal long-term memory (28%), concentration (13%), & language (11%)

Author/study	Sample	Time post-SAH	Measures	Outcome
Alfieri et al. (2008) *Prospective study*	N=30 SAH $\bar{x}$=41.7 years Non-Aneurysmal SAH	5-yrs	ZVNC, D2TA, WAIS-III (DS), WASI (BD, MR), RAVLT, BVRT, RRT, TLT, ROCF, WCST (modified)	Sig ↓ in all cognitive domains ↓ in attention and memory
Cheng et al. (2006) *Prospective study*	N=37 Aneurysmal SAH $\bar{x}$ =46.2	1 day-5-yrs	WAIS-R (Arithmetic, DS, DSy), WMS-R (PC, VR), COWAT, TMT, MMSE	29.7% no cognition ↓ 70.3% ↓ attention, memory, executive 37.8% -1 deficit, 32.4% > 2 deficits
Wong et al.(2009) *Prospective study*	N=40 SAH	9-27-mnths	FAB, RBMT, ADAS-Cog	global cognition ↓ in 35% ↓ executive functioning 27.5% ↓ memory in 43.6%
Madureira et al. (2000) *Prospective study*	N=22 Perimesencephalic SAH $\bar{x}$=54 years	39-mnths	MMSE, LC, WFT, Alternating Sequences, Proverb Interpretation, RPM, WMS, CD, WAIS (BD, Information), Simple Arithmetic, temporal, spatial, personal orientation test	72% ↓ in at least 1 domain Most ↓ visual memory (39%), abstract reasoning (33%)
Haug et al. (2010) *Prospective study*	N=26 Aneurysmal SAH $\bar{x}$ =49 yrs	1-yr	GPT, WAIS-III (DSy, DS), D-KEFS (CWIT, TMT, COWAT, DFT, CWIT), CVLT, CVLT-II, ROCFT, WASI-R (vocabulary, Similarities, BD, Matrices)	Mild ↓ (53%) psychomotor, executive, attention & intellectual function Moderate-severe ↓ (47%) motor, verbal and visual memory
Vilkki et al. (2004) *Prospective study*	N=138 Aneurysmal SAH $\bar{x}$=49.7 yrs	1-yr	WAIS-R (DS, Similarities, BD), CFIT, Face Searching, Face Recognition, MBVRT, Word list learning	↓ cognition: attention, general intelligence, & memory

Table 1. (Continued)

Author/study	Sample	Time post-SAH	Measures	Outcome
Hütter & Gilsbach (1992) *Prospective study*	N=48	2.8-yrs	WIP, d2, LPS-LD, LPS-RV, IST-memory, Benton-test, Stroop Test, TT, WD	↓ cognition: concentration, logical thinking, spatial abilities, language, memory, attention
Author/Study	Sample	Time post-SAH	Measures	Outcomes
Change over time				
Ogden et al. (1993) *Prospective study*	N=89 SAH x̄=16-69 yrs	12 wks & 12-mnths	WAIS-R (Vocabulary, Similarities, Comprehension, DS, PC, BD, PA, DSy), RMT (Words, Faces), WMS (Associate Learning, LM), ROCFT, OSR (Form I), TT, NART, GNT, MTDDA, VNT, TMT, WCST (modified)	↓ attention, visuospatial construction, memory, psycho-motor speed, mental flexibility though improve across all domains at 12 months Most ↓verbal cognition & memory
Koivisto et al. (2000) *Longitudinal*	N= 109 SAH	3 mnths & 12-mnths	WAIS-R (Similarities, Vocabulary, DS, PC, BD), BNT, COWAT, WMS (LM, VR), ROCFT, Stroop Test, TMT	12 mths: ↓ performance in all domains
Haug et al. (2007) *Prospective study*	N=32 SAH x̄=54 yrs	3,6 & 12-mnths	GPT, WAIS-III (DS), CVLT-II, ROCFT, D-KEFS (DS), WASI-R (Similarities, BD), BNT-short version	Cognition still ↓ at 12 mths At *3 mnths - 6 mths* ↑ Motor functioning At *12 mnths* ↑ verbal memory, ↓ verbal intelligence, aphasia, psychomotor, motor & executive functioning, visuospatial No↑ in attention
Samra et al. (2007) *Longitudinal*	N=185 SAH N =45 Controls	3, 9 & 15-mnths	BVRT-R, COWAT, GPT, ROCFT, TMT, NART-R	SAH group: Cognitive↑ occurred over time cognition ↓:*3-months*=35.7%; *9-months*=

Author/study	Sample	Time post-SAH	Measures	Outcome
				25.8%; *15-months*= 23.3%
Controlled comparisons				
Chahal, Barker-Collo, & Feigin (2011) *Cross-sectional Population Base*	N= 27 SAH N= 27 Controls x̄=62 yrs	5- years	MRS, GDS-15, CVLT-II, WMS-III LM, WMS-R VPA, ROCF, BNT. COWAT, WAIS-III BD and MR, Bell's test, Trails A/B, Victoria Stroop, IVA-CPT	SAH ↓ versus controls though effect sizes small.↓ attention, speed, story recall, word recall after delay, visuoperceptual ability (MR), and language testSAH also sig more depresse↓ memory and language impact on functional outcomes.
Powell et al. (2004) *Cross sectional*	N=49 SAH N=49 Controls x̄=46 yrs	18-mnths	DS, COWAT, & test of prose recall	-*18-mths*: ↓ attention, verbal fluency & memory
Ravnik et al. (2006) *Cross sectional*	N=10 SAH N=10 Controls x̄= 55 yrs	41-mnths	WCST, TLT, WMAS (verbal span, list acquisition, list recall, visual span, faces, visual reproduction), Stroop Test, D2TA, CTT	Mild degree of long-term cognitive ↓ Most ↓:memory & executive functioning
Author/Study	Sample	Time post-SAH	Measures	Outcomes
Germanò et al. (1998) *Cross sectional*	N=20 SAH =20 Controls x̄= 45.4 years	1-yr	WMS-R (LM, VPA, VDR, DS), TPT, WAIS-R (DS), TT, COWAT, BVRT-revised	-No sig cognitive differences in SAH and controls
Hadjivassiliou et al. (2001) Prospective	N= 80 SAH =31 Controls	1-yr	NART, WAIS-R (Vocabulary, DS, Arithmetic, PA, BD), story recall, face recognition, drawing complex figure, CANTB (CBS, ID/ED test, TLT), BNT, test of form discrimination, TMT	-Sig ↓: IQ, memory, executive functions, language, visual perception, attention, as compared to controls

Table 1. (Continued)

Author/study	Sample	Time post-SAH	Measures	Outcome
Mavaddat et al. (1999) *Cross sectional*	N= 47 SAH =20 Control $\bar{x}$=51.5 yrs Aneurysmal	6-24 mnths	MMSE, CANTB	-83% SAH cognition ↓: verbal fluency, pattern recognition and spatial working memory

Note: ACoA=Anterior Communicating Artery; ADAS-cog=Cognitive subscale of Alzhiemer Disease Assessment Scale; BD=Block Design; BT=Benton Test; BNT=Boston Naming Test; BVRT-R=Boston Visual Retention Test-Revised; CANTAB=Cambridge Automated Neuropsychological Battery; CD=Clock Drawing; COWAT=Controlled Oral Word Association Test; CTT=Color Trail Test; CVLT-II=California Verbal Learning Test; CWIT=Color Word Interference Test; D2TA=D2 Test of Attention; DS=Digit Span; DSy=Digit Symbol; D-KEFS=Delis-Kaplan Executive Functional System; EHT=Edinburgh Handedness Test; FAB=Frontal Assessment Battery; FTT=Finger-Tapping Test; GDS-15= Geriatric Depression Scale 15 item; GPT=Grooved Pegboard Test; HWIE=Hamburg Wechsler Intelligence Examination; ID/ED shift test=Intradimensional/Extradimensional Shift Test; IST=Intelligenz Struktur Test; IQ=Intelligent Quotient; IVA-CPT= Integrated Visual and Auditory Continuous Performance test; LC=Letter Cancellation; LM=Logical memory; LPS-LD=Leistungsprüfsystem-Lugisches Denken; LPS-RV=Leistungsprüfsystem Röumliche Vorstellungsvermögen; MBVRT=Modified Benton Visual Retention Test; MCA= Middle Cerebral Artery; MMSE=Mini Mental State Examination; MWCST=Modified Wisconsin Card-Sorting Test; MR= Matrix reasoning; MRS= Modified Rankin Scale; PA=Picture Arrangements; PC=Picture Completion; RBMT=Rivermead Behavioural Memory Test; ROCFT=Rey-Osterreith Complex Figure Test; RPM=Ravens Progressive Matrices; RRT=Rey Recovery Test; NART=National Adult Reading Test; PA=Paired associates; RMT=Recognition Memory Test; TLT= Tower of London Test; TMT-Trail Making Test; TT=Token Test; VNT= Visual Neglect Test; VPA=Visual Pared Associates; VR=Visual Reproduction; WAIS-R/III=Wechsler Adult Intelligence Scale-Revised/ Third edition; WASI-R= Wechsler Abbreviated Scale of Intelligence-Revised; WD= Weiner Determinationsgerät; WIF=Wechsler Intelligenz Prüfung; WMS-R/III= Wechsler Memory Scale-Revised/version III; WCST= Wisconsin Card-Sorting Test.

Prevalence rates of mood disorders post-stroke vary across studies with reported rates of PSD ranging from 9% to 22.8% at 3-months (Kauhanen et al., 1999; Kim & Choi-Kwon, 2000), 16% at 18-months (Palomaki et al., 1999), and 19% at 3-years post-stroke (Åström et al., 1993). In a recent population based study, 25.8% of stroke survivors had PSD with 3.6% experiencing severe PSD (Chausson et al., 2010). Prevalence of PSA reportedly ranges from 11-28% at 3-years post-stroke (Åström, 1996; Burvill et al., 1995). High rates of comorbidity have been reported with 85% of people with PSA also experiencing PSD at 3-years post-stroke (Castillo, Schultz & Robinson, 1995; Castillo, Starkstein, Fedoroff & Price, 1993).

Regarding SAH, studies have shown an increased rate of depression as compared to controls (Berry et al., 1997; Tidswell, Dias, Sagar, Mayes & Battersby, 1995), and moderate to severe depression and anxiety is prevalent for a long period post-SAH (Alfieri et al., 2008; Hütter et al., 1995; Powell et al., 2002). Similar to other stroke subtypes, SAH depression prevalence rates vary at different time periods with 16% (anxiety) and 14% (depression) at 3-months, and 17% (anxiety) and 8.5% (depression) at 9-months (Powell et al., 2002), and 20% (depression) and 40% (anxiety) at 16-months (Morris, Wilson & Dunn, 2004). A recent long-term study reported that 32% of participants report anxiety and 23% report depression 2 to 4-years post SAH (Visser-Meily, Rhebergsen, Rinkel, van Zandvoort & Post, 2009).

Discrepancies in prevalence rates may be attributed to differences in sample characteristics, assessment methods, testing time periods, and definitions of depression and anxiety across studies (Hackett, Yapa, Parag & Anderson, 2005). Many studies suffer from methodological limitations including selection bias (e.g., excluding the young or old, severe cases, those with cognitive impairments) and assessing at inconsistent time intervals post-SAH. Although numerous studies have examined the presence of post-SAH anxiety and depression, only one was located which was long-term and population based. In this study (Chahal et al. 2011), SAH survivors were significantly more depressed than matched controls but did not report significantly more anxiety at 5 years post SAH. None of the controls in this study met criteria for possible depression, whereas 29.6% of SAH survivors met these criteria.

In long-term studies, no association has been found between post-SAH depression or anxiety and type of SAH (aneurymal vs non-aneurysmal; anterior communicating artery aneurysm vs other) (Hütter et al., 1995), severity of haemorrhage, or time between admission and surgery as assessed by standardised measures (Morris et al., 2004). However, in terms of clinical severity, Kreitschmann-Andermahr et al. (2007) reported that post-SAH depression was significantly related to Glasgow Outcome Scores.

Numerous studies have reported a significant association between post-SAH depression and cognitive impairments (Andersen et al., 1995; Berg et al., 2003; Mayer et al., 2002) with depressed individuals experiencing more cognitive deficits (House, Dennis, Warlow, Hawton & Molyneux, 1990; Rasquin et al., 2005; Srikanth et al., 2006). Indeed, cognitive complaints such as reduced processing speed, and problems with memory and attention are common post-SAH and are strongly associated with depression (Passier et al., 2010). Alfieri et al. (2008) note that depression is associated with reduced attention in SAH survivors at 1-year.

Long Term Activity and Participation (HRQoL) in SAH Survivors

With case-fatality after SAH reducing over the past 3 decades and the relatively young age of onset of SAH at around 55 years, (Lovelock, Rinkel, & Rothwell, 2010), there is an increased prevalence of survivors of SAH with a good life expectancy. While the focus of medical attention after SAH is mainly on neurological deficits; psychological, psychosocial and cognitive impairment after SAH can contribute to and negatively affect health-related quality of life (HRQoL). HRQoL refers to how "health impacts on an individual's ability to function and his or her perceived well-being in physical, mental and social domains of life", and can be framed within the ICF (Coons, Rao, Keininger, & Hays, 2000) (p. 28). Activity limitation refers to difficulties in executing activities, while participation limitation refers to difficulties with involvement, such as returning to work (Passier, Visser-Meily, Rinkel, Lindeman, & Post, 2013) Reduced HRQoL can be present despite functional independence (Passier et al., 2013) and impacts long-term day-to-day activity, participation and (Al-Khindi, Macdonald, & Schweizer, 2010). Often the greatest impact of SAH on HRQoL occurs in the home or community setting and in the absence of medical management (He & Mack, 2014). Thus, HRQoL is an important outcome to evaluate due to its impact on activity and participation, and to inform rehabilitation and medical management. HRQoL evaluation also has the potential to identify relevant predictors of reduced HRQOL to in order to inform ways to minimise their impact.

Studies of long-term HRQoL in SAH have used varying measures including the EuroQol Instrument (EQ5D) and the EuroQol Visual Analogue scale (EQ VAS), the Sickness Impact Profile (SIP) and the Medical Outcomes Study 36-Item Short Form (SF-36), while follow-up intervals varied from a few months to several years (Coons et al., 2000; Rinkel & Algra, 2011). The most commonly affected domains of HRQoL in SAH appear to be emotional, social and physical functioning (Al-Khindi et al., 2010). HRQoL measures at 6 months to one year after SAH were found to be reduced after SAH and up to one year compared to the normal population, however improvements in HRQoL of 12-14% were seen from three months onwards compared the time of hospital discharge (Meyer et al., 2010). Worse HRQoL in this study was associated with female gender, severe SAH, functional disability, depression, lower education levels and the lack of a stable partnership. Worse HRQoL with the EQ5D was also found in a Swedish study at 9 months after SAH with the largest difference found in the usual activities domain (Ronne-Engström, Enblad, & Lundström, 2011). Interestingly, mood problems tended to decrease after the age of 40 years. In a study looking at whether there were any differences between surgically treated versus endovascularly treated patients with good outcome, no differences in HRQoL were found at 1 year between the two groups, however psychological changes were reported in general in both groups, with lower quality of life in the areas of intimate relationship and health (Preiss et al., 2012). A cross-sectional study of patients 2-4 years after SAH found the HRQoL score was at satisfactory level, but a divergence was seen with lower scores in the emotional and social domains compared to the physical domain (Visser-Meily, Rhebergen, Rinkel, Van Zandvoort, & Post, 2009). Personality characteristics and psychological symptoms were strongly correlated to a reduced HRQoL score in this study, including mood problems, fatigue, and cognitive problems. These findings suggest an increased prevalence of these predictors of worse HRQoL after SAH as shown in a study where SAH patients had increased mood disturbance, subtle cognitive impairment, and reduced independence and social participation at 3 and 9months after SAH compared to the normal population (Powell, Kitchen, Heslin, & Greenwood, 2002). SAH was shown to have marked effect of on employment status at 2-4 years with only 35% of those previously employed resuming work completely (Passier, Anne Visser-Meily, Rinkel, Lindeman, & Post, 2011). Additionally, in terms of life satisfaction, only around 50% were satisfied with their employment situation and sexual life. Fatigue may also be an important contributor to reduced HRQoL; found to be present 1 year after SAH in 71% of patients, and associated with increased physical and cognitive problems (Passier, Post, et al., 2011).

A much longer-term follow-up (median follow-up 10.8 years) of SAH patients treated with either clipping or coiling found that the EQ-5D index and the EQ5D VAS were similar to that of the normal population, with 88% of people living at home and 63% returning to work after SAH (Malmivaara, Juvela, Hernesniemi, Lappalainen, & Siironen, 2012). However, the study excluded those over 75 years which may have resulted in a higher QoL index. Functional outcome as measured with the modified Rankin Scale (mRS) and overall quality of life scores with the SF-36 and VAS had improved in the majority of patients at 5 years compared to 4 months after SAH and had continued to improve at 12.5 years (Greebe, Rinkel, Hop, Visser-Meily, & Algra, 2010). In contrast, a study in Stockholm that also followed up patients after 10 years found that SAH patients had significantly more problems in 4 of the 5 domains of the EQ-5D compared to the general population (von Vogelsang, Burstrom, Wengstrom, Svensson, & Forsberg, 2013). The worst outcomes were seen in those with worse GCS scores at discharge, those with comorbidities and those with low perception of recovery. Similarly, it has been found that HRQOL was reduced 10 years after SAH to a similar level as 1, 2 and 5 years (Kapapa, Woischneck, & Tjahjadi, 2014), in a study that included a survey of proxies which corroborated patient findings.

Several studies have examined HRQoL and its associated predictors at varying times after SAH in order to determine their impact on SAH outcomes. Reduced HRQoL was associated with depression in the first 12 months after SAH (Kreiter et al., 2013). Cognitive problems and a passive coping style at 3 months as well as female gender were associated with reduced HRQoL as measured by the Stroke Specific Quality of life Scale (SS-QoL) (Passier et al., 2012). Fear of recurrence or that new aneurysms can develop and existing aneurysms can grow after the initial SAH are factors which have been found to worsen HRQoL in both patients and their significant others (Covey, Noble, & Schenk, 2013; Rinkel & Algra, 2011). It is suggested that this fear may lead significant others to be overprotective and limit patients' activities. Interestingly a meta-analysis of predictors of poor HRQoL found that only physical disability had a notable impact on HRQoL, whereas traditional factors such as age, sex, neurological deficit, bleed severity, physical disability, and cognitive impairment were found not to be significant predictors of HRQoL (Noble & Schenk, 2010). This is unlike most other studies where the mental health component of the HRQoL was a more significant predictor than the physical component. The authors suggested that a large proportion of the variance of patients' HRQoL remains unexplained. One of the predictors that may contribute to this variance was suggested to be posttraumatic stress disorder (PSTD). PTSD as a result of the traumatic experience of SAH has also been linked with reduced quality of life after SAH. PTSD was found in 37% of patients compared to an expected prevalence on 8% in the general population and that it is a major determinant of psychosocial outcome (Noble et al., 2008). This suggests that future studies need to explore novel predictors of HRQoL outcome after SAH that may have a stronger association with outcomes.

In summary, HRQoL is an important outcome to assess after SAH, in order to track temporal changes in recovery and to more accurately inform treatment and rehabilitation. While physical rehabilitation tends to take precedence, psychosocial and mental health outcomes are often not assessed and addressed, and even less so in the holistic context of the patient, family, work, social life and other environmental contributors of HRQoL. A cyclic construct has been proposed for long-term recovery after SAH where physical, mental and social impairment may contribute to unemployment, which then contributes in turn to a further decline in physical, mental an social domains (He & Mack, 2014). The direction and interplay of these factors can either have a positive or negative impact on HRQoL in the long-term and understanding these processes will aid healthcare professionals to develop strategies to optimise outcomes for both patients, their families after SAH (He & Mack, 2014).

Discussion

Though constituting only a small proportion of incident stroke cases, SAH has a higher case fatality than other stroke types. As outcomes for those who survive beyond 28-days tend to change overtime, studying long-term outcomes of SAH is important in order to better understand its natural course and the impact of various management strategies. It is also important to study these outcomes in a population-based manner in order that the full scope of outcomes may be captured, yet there are few population based studies of SAH survivors beyond 12 months and even fewer examine wider outcomes such as neuropsychological outcomes, quality of life and mood. In this chapter we reviewed the existing literature on long-term (> 12 months) health outcomes of SAH with a focus on these less evidenced outcomes and placing these in the context of the WHO models of health.

The findings reviewed here suggest that SAH survivors who make a good overall recovery or do well on global outcome measures (e.g., Glasgow

Outcome Scale Score) still exhibit cognitive deficits. While the data on these outcomes is quite variable, the most commonly reported area of continuing deficit is in both verbal and visual memory. The presence of cognitive impairments post-SAH is linked to presence of mood disorders, particularly depression. Numerous studies have reported a significant association between post-SAH depression and cognitive impairments.

Depression is more common in the long term post-SAH when compared to controls with prevalence rates of 14% rising 20% at 16-months (Morris, Wilson & Dunn, 2004), and 23% report at 2 to 4-years post SAH (Visser-Meily, Rhebergsen, Rinkel, van Zandvoort & Post, 2009). Anxiety is also reported to occur post-SAH, with the one long-term population based study to report on anxiety and depression (Chahal et al. 2011), finding that 29.6% of SAH survivors met criteria for possible depression as compared to none of the matched controls, and that SAH survivors did not report significantly more anxiety than controls at 5 years post SAH. As might be expected Kreitschmann-Andermahr et al. (2007) reported that post-SAH depression was significantly related to SAH severity (as indicated by Glasgow Outcome Scores).

While the focus of medical attention after SAH is mainly on neurological deficits, psychological, psychosocial and cognitive impairment after SAH can contribute to and negatively affect health-related quality of life (HRQoL). Indeed, the literature reviewed here indicates that cognitive problems, depression and passive coping style, and fear of recurrence are modifiable factors which have been linked to the wider HRQoL outcomes after SAH.

The interconnectedness of these various outcomes is in line with the WHO models of health described at the outset of this chapter, and also makes intuitive sense if one considers a typical SAH survivor. Such an individual has experienced traumatic and unexpected medical emergency which has most likely led to a hospital stay, surgery, and a disruption in everyday activities upon return home. This scenario would, understandably, lead to feelings of fear that the experience might be repeated, as well as depressed mood as the individual comes to term with resultant loss of abilities, and changes in activities and expectations in day to day life. These emotional reactions might contribute to or be exacerbated by difficulties in cognition, such as reduced memory abilities. Taken together, the individual would then be expected to report a reduction in his or her overall quality of life.

Of note here is that these factors are modifiable through psychological and cognitive rehabilitation interventions. In their review of evidence for cognitive rehabilitation Cicerone and colleagues (2010) conclude that there is substantial evidence to support both targeted interventions for cognitive abilities such as attention and memory, as well as for comprehensive-holistic neuropsychological rehabilitation after TBI. Thus, while it may not be possible to improve upon neurological outcomes post-SAH, there remains a window of opportunity to improve life outcomes through intervention.

Conclusion

We have reviewed research findings on long term (>12 months) health outcomes of SAH within the WHO model of health, and including population based studies. Although the incidence of SAH is much lower than the other stroke types, it case fatality is much higher. The review demonstrated that long term SAH survivors demonstrate cognitive difficulties, particularly in verbal and visual memory. Depression was more common than controls and is likely exacerbates cognitive impairments. There was evidence that depression is linked to severity of SAH.

References

Albrecht, G., Sleeman, K., & Bury, M. (2001). *Handbook of Disability Studies.* London: Sage Publications.

Alfieri, A., Unterhuber, V., Pircher, M., Schwarz, A. Gazzeri, R., Reinert, M., et al. (2008). Psychosocial and neurocognitive performance after spontaneous nonaneurysmal subarachnoid hemorrhage related to the APOE-ε4 genotype: A prospective 5-year follow-up study. *Journal of Neurosurgery, 109,* 1019-1026.

Algurén, B., Lundgren-Nilsson, A., & Sunnerhagen, K.S. (2010). Functioning of stroke survivors: A validation of the ICF core set for stroke in Sweden. *Disability and Rehabilitation, 32*(7), 551-559.

Al-Khindi, T., Macdonald, R. L., & Schweizer, T. A. (2010). Cognitive and functional outcome after aneurysmal subarachnoid hemorrhage *Stroke, 41*(8), e519-536

Andersen, G.,Vestergaard, K., Ingemann-Nielsen M., & Lauritzen, L. (1995). Risk factors for post-stroke depression. *Acta Psychiatrica Scandinavica, 92,* 193-198.

Åström, M. (1996). Generalized anxiety disorder in stroke patients: A 3-year longitudinal study. *Stroke, 27,* 270-275.

Åström, M., Adolfsson, R., & Asplund, K. (1993). Major depression in stroke patients: A 3-year longitudinal study. *Stroke, 24,* 976-982.

Badley, E. (1993). An introduction to the concepts and classification of the international classification of impairments, disabilities, and handicaps. *Disability and Rehabilitation, 15*(4), 161-178.

Ballard, C., Rowan, E., Stepehns, S., Kalaria, R., & Kenny, R. (2003). Prospective follow up study between 3 and 15 months after stroke: Improvements and decline in cognitive functioning among dementia free stroke survivours below 75 years of age. *Stroke , 34,* 2440-2444.

Barker-Collo, S. (2007). Depression and anxiety 3 months post stroke: Prevalence and correlates. *Archives of Clinical Neuropsychology, 22*(4), 519-531.

Berg, A., Palomäki, H., Lehtihalmes, M., Lönnqvist, J., & Kaste, M. (2003). Poststroke depression: An 18-month follow-up. *Stroke, 43,* 138-143.

Berry, E., Jones, R.A.C., West, C.G.H., & Brown, J.D.K. (1997). Outcome of subarachnoid hemorrhage: an anlysis of surgical variables, cognitive and emotional sequelae related to SPECT scanning. *British Journal of Neurosurgery, 11*(5), 378-387.

Burvill, P.W., Johnson, G.A., Jamrozik, C.S., Anderson, C.S., Stewart-Wynne, E.G., & Chakera, T.M.H. (1995). Anxiety disorders after stroke: Results from the Perth Community Stroke Study. *British Journal of Psychiatry, 166*, 328-332.

Castillo, C. S., Schultz, S. K., & Robinson, R. (1995). Clinical correlates of early onset and late-onset poststroke generalised anxiety. *American Journal of Psychiatry, 152*(8), 1174-1181.

Castillo, C. S., Starkstein, S. E., Fedoroff, J. P., & Price, T. R. (1993). Generalized anxiety disorder after stroke. *Journal of Nervous & Mental Disease, 181*(2), 100-106.

Chahal, N., Barker-Collo, S. & Feigin, V. Neuropsychological and functional outcomes of 5-year subarachnoid hemorrhage survivors: Comparison to matched controls. *Neuroepidemiology*, 37, 31-38.

Chausson, N., Olindo, S., Cabre, P., Saint-Vil, M., & Smadja, D. (2010). Five year outcomes of a stroke cohort in Martinique French West indies: Edute realisee en Martinique et centree sut l'incedence des accidents vasculaire cerebraux, Part 2. *Stroke, 41*(5), 594-599.

Cheng, H., Shi, J., & Zhou, M. (2006). Cognitive assessment in Chinese patients with aneurysmal subarachnoid hemorrhage. *Behavioural Neurology, 17,* 117-120.

Cicerone KD, Langenbahn DM, Braden C, Malec JF, Kalmar K, Fraas M, Felicetti T, Laatsch L, Harley JP, Bergquist T, Azulay J, Cantor J, Ashman T. (2010) Evidence-based cognitive rehabilitation: updated review of the literature from 2003 through 2008. *Archives of Physical Medicine and Rehabilitation,* 92 (4), 519-530.

Cieza A., Geyh, S., Chatterji, S., Kostanjsek, N., Üstün, B.T., & Stucki, G. (2006). Identification of candidate categories of the International Classification of Functioning Disability and Health (ICF) for a generic ICF core set based on regression modelling. *BMC Medical Research Methodology, 6*(36), 1-16.

Coons, S. J., Rao, S., Keininger, D. L., & Hays, R. D. (2000). A comparative review of generic quality-of-life instruments. *PharmacoEconomics, 17*(1), 13-35.

Covey, J., Noble, A. J., & Schenk, T. (2013). Family and friends' fears of recurrence: impact on the patient's recovery after subarachnoid hemorrhage. *Journal of Neurosurgery, 119*(4), 948-954.

Egge., A., Waterloo., K., Sjøholm., H., Ingebrigtsen, T., Forsdahl., S., Jacobsen, E.A., et al. (2004). Outcome 1 year after aneurysmal subarachnoid hemorrhage: Relation between cognitive performance and neuroimaging. *Acta Neurologica Scandinavica, 112,* 76-80.

Ewert, T., Allen, D.D., Wislon, M., Üstün, B., & Stucki, G. (2010). Validation of the international classification of functioning disability and health framework using multidimensional item response modelling. *Disability and Rehabilitation, 32*(17), 1397-1405.

Frazer, D., Ahuja, A., Watkins, L., & Cipolotti, L. (2007). Coiling versus clipping for the treatment of aneurysmal subarachnoid hemorrhage: A longitudinal investigation into cognitive outcome. *Neurosurgery, 60,* 434-442.

Fougeyrollas, P. (1995). Documenting environmental factors for preventing the handicap creation process: Quebec contributions relating to ICIDH and social participation of people with functional differences. *Disability and Rehabilitation, 17*(3-4), 145-153.

Germanò, A., Caruso, G., Caffo, M., Cacciola, F., Belvedere, M., Tisano, A., et al. (1998). Does subarachnoid blood extravasation *per se* induce long-term neuropsychological and cognitive alterations? *Acta Neurochirurgica, 140,* 805-812.

Goodwin, R.D., & Devanand, D.P. (2008). Stroke, depression, and functional health outcomes among adults in the community. *Journal of Geriatric Psychiatry, 21*(1), 41-46.

Gray, D.B., & Hendershot, G.E. (2000). The ICIDH-2: Developments for a new era of outcomes research. *Archives of Physical and Medical Rehabilitation, 81*(Suppl. 2), 10-14.

Greebe, P., Rinkel, G. J. E., Hop, J. W., Visser-Meily, J. M. A., & Algra, A. (2010). Functional outcome and quality of life 5 and 12.5 years after aneurysmal subarachnoid hemorrhage. *Journal of Neurology, 257*(12), 2059-2064.

Grill, E., Ewert, T., Chatterji, S., Kostanjsek, N., & Stucki, G. (2005). ICF core sets development for the acute hospital and early post-acute rehabilitation facilities. *Disability and Rehabilitation, 27*(7-8), 361-366.

Haacke, C., Althaus, A., Spottke, A., Siebert, U., Back, T., & Dodel, R. (2006). Long-term outcome after stroke: Evaluating health-related quality of life using utility measurements. *Stroke, 37,* 193-198.

Hackett, M.L., Duncan, J.R., Anderson, C.S., Broad, J.B., & Bonita, R. (2000). Health-related quality of life among long-term survivors of stroke: Results from the Auckland Stroke Study, 1991-1992. *Stroke, 31,* 440-447.

Hackett, M.L., Yapa, C., Parag, V., & Anderson, C.S. (2005). Frequency of depression after stroke: A systematic review of observational studies. *Stroke, 36,* 130-1340.

Hadjivassiliou, M., Tooth, C.L., Romanowski, C.A.J., Byrne, J., Battersby, R.D.E., Oxbury, S., et al. (2001). Cognitive outcome and structural damage after clipping and coiling. *Neurology, 56,* 1672-1677.

Haug, T., Sorteberg, A., Finset., A.., Lindegaard, K., Lundar, T., & Sorteberg, W. (2010). Cognitive functioning and health related quality of life 1 year after aneurysmal subarachnoid hemorrhage in preoperative comotose patients (Hunt and Hess Grade V patients). *Neurosurgery, 66*(3), 475-485.

Haug, T., Sorteberg, A., Sorteberg, W., Lindegaard, K., Lundar, T., & Finset., A. (2007). Cognitive outcome after aneurysmal subarachnoid hemorrhage: Time course of recovery and relationship to clinical, radiological, and management parameters. *Neurosurgery, 60,* 649-657.

Haug, T., Sorteberg, A., Sorteberg, W., Lindegaard, K., Lundar, T., & Finset., A. (2009). Cognitive function and health related quality of life after rupture of an aneurysm on the anterior communicating artery versus middle cerebral artery. *British Journal of Neurosurgey, 23*(5), 507-515.

He, S., & Mack, W. J. (2014). Health-related quality of life after aneurysmal subarachnoid hemorrhage: interplay between physical, cognitive, and emotional factors [Comment]. *World Neurosurgery, 81*(1), 37-39.

Hedlund, M., Zetterling, M., Ronne-Engstrom, E., Ekselius L., & Carlsson, M. (2010). Perceived recovery after aneurysmal subarachnoid hemorrhage in individuals with or without depression. *Journal of Clinical Nursing, 19,* 1578-1587.

Hop, J.W., Rinkel, G.J.E., Algra, A., & van Gijn, J. (1997). Case-fatality rates and functional outcome after subarachnoid hemorrhage. *Stroke, 28,* 660-664.

House, A., Dennis, M., Warlow, C., Hawton, K., & Molyneux, A. (1990). The relationship between intellectual impairment and mood disorder in the first year aftre stroke. *Psychological Medicine, 20,* 805-814.

Hütter, B. O, & Gilsabch, J. M. (1992). Cognitive deficits after rupture and early repair of anterior communicating artery aneurysms. *Acta Neurochirurgica, 116,* 6-13.

Hütter, B.O., & Gilsabch, J.M. (1993). Which neuropsychological deficits are hidden behind a good outcome (Glasgow=I) after aneurysmal subarachnoid hemorrhage? *Neurosurgery, 33*(6), 999-1006.

Hütter, B.O, & Gilsabch, J.M., & Kreitschmann-Andermahr, I. (1995). Quality of life and cognitive deficits after subarachnoid hemorrhage. *British Journal of Neurosurgery, 9,* 465-475.

Jette, J.M. (2006). Towards a common language for function, disability, and health. *Physical Therapy, 86*(5), 726-734.

Kapapa, T., Woischneck, D., & Tjahjadi, M. (2014). Long-term health-related quality of life after spontaneous nontraumatic subarachnoid hemorrhage: self and proxy reports in a 10-year period. *World Neurosurgery, 81*(1), 105-109

Kauhanen, H., Korpelainen, J.T., Hiltunen, P., Brusin, E., Mononen, H., Määttä, R., et al. (1999). Poststroke depression correlates with cognitive impairment and neurological deficits. *Stroke, 30,* 1875-1880.

Kim, J., & Choi-Kwon, S. (2000). Poststroke depressionand emotional incontinence: Correlation with lesion location. *Neurology, 54*(9), 1805-1810.

Koivisto, T., Vanninen, R.V., Hurskainen, H., Saari, T., Hernesniemi, J., & Vapalahti. (2000). Outcomes of early endovascular versus surgical treatment of ruptured carebral aneurysms: A prospective randomised study. *Stroke, 31,* 2369-2377.

Kreiter, K. T., Rosengart, A. J., Claassen, J., Fitzsimmons, B. F., Peery, S., Du, Y. E., ... Mayer, S. A. (2013). Depressed mood and quality of life after subarachnoid hemorrhage *Journal of the Neurological Sciences, 335*(1-2), 64-71.

Kreitschmann-Andermahr, I., Poll, I., Hutter, B., Reineke, A., Kristes, S., Gisbach., et al. (2007). Quality of life and psychiatric sequelae following aneurismal subarachnoid hemorrhage: does neuroendocrine dysfunction play a role? *Clinical Endocrinology, 66,* 833-837.

Lezak, M. D., Howieson, D. B., & Loring, D. W. (2004). *Neuropsychological assessment* (4th ed.). New York, NY: Oxford University Press.

Longstreth, W.T., Koepsell, T.D., Yerby, M.S., & van Belle, G. (1985). Risk factors for subarachnoid hemorrhage. *Stroke, 16,* 377-385.

Lovelock, C. E., Rinkel, G. J. E., & Rothwell, P. M. (2010). Time trends in outcome of subarachnoid hemorrhage: Population-based study and systematic review. *Neurology, 74*(19), 1494-1501.

Madureira, S., Canhão, P., Guerreiro, M., & Ferro, J.M. (2000). Cognitive and emotional consequences of periencephalic subarachnoid hemorrhage. *Journal of Neurology, 415,* 862-867.

Malmivaara, K., Juvela, S., Hernesniemi, J., Lappalainen, J., & Siironen, J. (2012). Health-related quality of life and cost-effectiveness of treatment in subarachnoid hemorrhage. *European Journal of Neurology, 19*(11), 1455-1461.

Mavaddat, N., Sahakian, B.J., Hutchinson, P.J.A., & Kirkpatrick, P.J. (1999). Cognition following subarachnoid hemorrhage from anterior communicating artery aneurysm: Relation to timing of surgery. *Journal of Neurosurgery, 91,* 402-407.

Mayer, S.A., Kreiter, K.T., Copeland, D., Bernardini, G.L., Bates, J.E., Peery, S., et al. (2002). Global and domain specific cognitive impairment and outcome after subarachnoid hemorrhage. *Neurology, 59,* 1750-1758.

Meyer, B., Ringel, F., Winter, Y., Spottke, A., Gharevi, N., Dams, J., ... Dodel, R. (2010). Health-related quality of life in patients with subarachnoid hemorrhage. *Cerebrovascular Diseases, 30*(4), 423-431.

Mocco, J., Ransom, E.R., Komotar, R.J., Sergot, P.B., Ostapkovich, N., Schmidt, J.M., et al. (2006,). Long-term domain specific improvement following poor grade aneurysmal subarachniod hemorrhage. *Journal of Neurology, 253,* 1278-1284.

Morris, P.G., Wilson, J.T. L., & Dunn, L. (2004). Anxiety and depression after spontaneous subarachnoid hemorrhage. *Neurosurgery, 54,* 47-54.

Noble, A. J., Baisch, S., Mendelow, A. D., Allen, L., Kane, P., & Schenk, T. (2008). Posttraumatic stress disorder explains reduced quality of life in subarachnoid hemorrhage patients in both the short and long term. *Neurosurgery, 63*(6), 1095-1104.

Noble, A. J., & Schenk, T. (2010). Which variables help explain the poor health-related quality of life after subarachnoid hemorrhage? A meta-analysis. *Neurosurgery, 66*(4), 772-783

Ogden, J.A., Levin, P.L., & Mee, E.W. (1990). Long-term neuropsychological and psychosocial effects of subarachnoid hemorrhage. *Neuropsychiatry, Neuropsychology, and Behavioral Neurology, 3*(4), 260-274.

Ogden, J.A., Mee, E., & Henning, M. (1993). A prospective study of impairment of cognition and memory and recovery after subarachnoid hemorrhage. *Neurosurgery, 33*(4), 572-587.

Ogden, J.A., Utley,T., & Mee, E.W. (1997). Neurological and Psychosocial outcome 4 to 7 years after subarachnoid hemorrhage. *Neurosurgery, 41*(1), 25-34.

Passier, P. E. C. A., Anne Visser-Meily, J. M. A., Rinkel, G. J. E., Lindeman, E., & Post, M. W. M. (2011). Life satisfaction and return to work after aneurysmal subarachnoid hemorrhage. *Journal of Stroke and Cerebrovascular Diseases, 20*(4), 324-329.

Passier, P.E.C.A., Visser-Meily, J.M.A., van Zandvoort, M.J.E., Post, M.W.M., Rinkel., G.J.E., & van Heugten, C. (2010). Prevalence and detreminants of cognitive complaints after aneurysmal subarachnoid hemorrhage. *Cerbrovascular Disease, 29,* 557-563.

Passier, P. E. C. A., Visser-Meily, J. M. A., Rinkel, G. J. E., Lindeman, E., & Post, M. W. M. (2013). Determinants of health-related quality of life after aneurysmal subarachnoid hemorrhage: A systematic review. *Quality of Life Research, 22*(5), 1027-1043.

Passier, P. E. C. A., Post, M. W. M., Van Zandvoort, M. J. E., Rinkel, G. J. E., Lindeman, E., & Visser-Meily, J. M. A. (2011). Predicting fatigue 1 year after aneurysmal subarachnoid hemorrhage. *Journal of Neurology, 258*(6), 1091-1097.

Passier, P. E. C. A., Visser-Meily, J. M. A., van Zandvoort, M. J. E., Rinkel, G. J. E., Lindeman, E., & Post, M. W. M. (2012). Predictors of long-term health-related quality of life in patients with aneurysmal subarachnoid hemorrhage. *Neurorehabilitation, 30*(2), 137-145.

Powell, J., Kitchen, N., Heslin, J., & Greenwood, R. (2002). Psychosocial outcomes at three and nine months after good neurological recovery from aneurysmal subarachnoid hemorrhage: predictors and prognosis. *Journal of Neurology, Neurosurgery & Psychiatry, 72*(6), 772-781.

Preiss, M., Netuka, D., Koblihova, J., Bernardova, L., Charvat, F., Kratochvilova, D., & Benes, V. (2012). Quality of life 1 year after aneurysmal subarachnoid hemorrhage in good outcome patients treated by clipping or coiling. *Journal of Neurological Surgery, Part A: Central European Neurosurgery, 73*(4), 217-223.

Powell, J., Kitchen, N., Heslin, J., & Greenwood, R. (2002). Psychosocial outcomes at three and nine months after good neurological recovery from aneurismal subarachnoid hemorrhage: Predictors and prognosis. *Journal of Neurology, Neurosurgery and Psychiatry, 72,* 772-781.

Powell, J., Kitchen, N., Heslin, J., & Greenwood, R. (2004). Psychosocial outcomes at 18 months after good neurological recovery from aneurismal subarachnoid hemorrhage. *Journal of Neurology, Neurosurgery, and Psychiatry, 75,* 1119-1124.

Rasquin, S., Lodder, J., & Verhey, F. (2005). The association between psychiatric and cognitive symptoms after stroke: A prospective study. *Cervebrovascular Disease, 19,* 309-316.

Ravnik., J., Starovasnik, B., Šešok, S., Pirtošek, Z., Švigelj, V., Bunc, G., & Bošnjak., R. (2006). Long-term cognitive deficits in patients with good outcomes after aneurysmal subarachnoid hemorrhage from anterior communicating artery. *Croatian Medical Journal, 47,* 253-263.

Rinkel, G. J. E., & Algra, A. (2011). Long-term outcomes of patients with aneurysmal subarachnoid hemorrhage. *Lancet Neurology, 10*(4), 349-356.

Rosamond, W., Katherine, F., Friday, G., Furie, K., Go, A., Greenlund, K., et al. (2007). Heart disease and stroke statistics-2007 update: A report from the American Heart association Statistics committee and stroke statistics subcommittee. *Circulation, 115,* 69-171.

Ronne-Engström, E., Enblad, P., & Lundström, E. (2011). Outcome after spontaneous subarachnoid hemorrhage measured with the EQ-5D. *Stroke, 42*(11), 3284-3286.

Saciri, B.M., & Kos, N. (2002). Aneurysmal subarachnoid hemorrhage: Outcomes of early rehabilitation after surgical repair of ruptured intracranial aneurysms. *Journal of Neurology, Neurosurgery and Psychiatry, 72,* 334-337.

Samra, S.K., Giordani, B., Caveney, A.F., Clarke, W.R., Scott, P.A., Anderson, S., et al. (2007). Recovery of cognitive function after surgery for aneurysmal subarachnoid hemorrhage. *Stroke, 38,* 1864-1872.

Scharbrodt, W., Stein, M., Schreiber, V., Böker, D., & Oertel., M.F. (2009). The prediction of long-term outcome after subarachnoid hemorrhage as measured by the short form-36 health survey. *Journal of Clinical Neuroscience, 16,* 1409-1413.

Srikanth, V.K., Thrift, A., Saling, M.M., Anderson, J.F.I., Dewey, H.M., Macdonell, R.A.L., et al. (2003). Increased risk of cognitive impairment 3 months after mild to moderate first-ever stroke: A community base prospective study of nonaphasic English-speaking survivors. *Stroke, 34,* 1136-1143.

Srikanth, V.K., Quinn, S.J., Donnan, G.A., Saling, M.M., & Thrift, AG. (2006). Long-term cognitive transitions, rates of cognitive change, and predictors of incident dementia in a population-based first-ever stroke cohort. *Stroke, 37,* 2479-2483.

Starrost, K., Geyh, S., Trautwein, A., Grunow, J., Ceballos-Baumann, A., Prosigel, M., et al., (2008). Inter-rater relaibility of the Extended ICF Core Set for stroke applied by physical therapists. *Physical Therpay , 88*(7), 841-851.

Strong, K., Mathers, C., & Bonita, R. (2007). Preventing stroke: Saving lives around the world. *The Lancet Neurology, 6,* 182-187.

Sturm, J.W., Donnan, G.A., Dewey, H.M., Macdonell, R.A.L., Gilligan, A.K., Srikanth, V., et al. (2004). Quality of life after stroke: The North East Melbourne Stroke Incidence Study (NEMESIS). *Stroke, 35,* 2340-2345.

Stucki, G. (2005). International classification of functioning disability and health: A promising framework and classification for rehabilitation medicine. *American Journal of Physical Medicine and Rehabilitation , 84,* 733-740.

Stucki, G., Cieza A., & Melvin, J. (2007). The international classification of functioning, disability and health: A unifying model for the conceptual description of the rehabilitation strategy. *Journal of Rehabilitation Medicine, 39,* 279-285.

Thrift, A., Dewey, H., Macdonell, R., McNeil, J., & Donnan, G. (2001). Incidence of the major stroke subtypes: Initial findings from the North East Melbourne Stroke Incidence Study (NEMESIS). *Stroke, 32,* 1732-1738.

Tidswell, P., Dias, P.S., Sagar, H.J., Mayes, A., & Buttersby, R.D. (1995). Cognitive outcome after aneurysm rupture: Relationship to aneurysm site and preoperative complications. *Neurology, 45,* 875-882.

Townend, B.S., Whyte, S., Desborough, T., Crimmins, D., Markus, R., Levi, C., et al. (2007). Longitudinal prevalence and determinants of early mood disorder post-stroke. *Journal of Clinical Neuroscience, 81*(7), 881-887.

Uski, T.K., Lilja, Å., Säveland, H., Ekman, R., Sonesson, B., & Brandt, L. (2000). Cognitive functioning and cerebrospinal fluid concentrations of neuropeptides for patients with good neurological outcomes after aneurysmal subarachnoid hemorrhage. *Neurosurgery, 47,* 812-818.

Üstün, B., Chatterji, S., & Kostanjsek, N. (2004). Comments from WHO for the Journal of Rehabilitation Medicine special supplement on ICF core sets. *Journal of Rehabilitation Medicine, 44*, 7-8.

Vilkki, J. S., Juvela, S., Siironen, J., Ilvonen, T., Varis, J., & Porras, M. (2004). Relationship of local infarctions to cognitive and psychosocial impairments after aneurysmal subarachnoid hemorrhage. *Neurosurgery, 55,* 790-803.

Visser-Meily, J.M.A., Rhebergsen, M.L., Rinkel, G.J.E., van Zandvoort, M. J., & Post, M.W.M. (2009). Long-term health-related quality of life after aneurysmal subarachnoid hemorrhage: Relationship with psychological symptoms and ersonality characteristics. *Stroke, 40,* 1526-1529.

von Vogelsang, A.-C., Burstrom, K., Wengstrom, Y., Svensson, M., & Forsberg, C. (2013). Health-related quality of life 10 years after intracranial aneurysm rupture: a retrospective cohort study using EQ-5D. *Neurosurgery, 72*(3), 397-405

Wilkinson, P.R., Wolfe, C.D.A., Warburton, F.G., Rudd, A.G., Howards, R.S., Ross-Russell, R.W., et al. (1997). A long-term follow-up of stroke patients. *Stroke, 28,* 507-512.

Wong, G.K.C., Wong, R., Mok, V.C.T., Fan, D.S.P., Leung, G., Wong, A., et al. (2009). Clinical study on cognitive dysfunction after spontaneous subarachnoid hemorrhage: Patient profiles and relationship to cholinergic dysfunction. *Acta Neurochirurgica, 151,* 1601-1607.

World Health Organisation. (1980). *International classification of Impairments, Disabilities and Handicap: A manual of classification relating to consequences of disease.* Geneva, Switzerland: World Health Organisation.

World Health Organisation. (2001). *International classification of Functioning, Disability and Handicap.* Geneva, Switzerland: World Health Organisation.

Whyte, E.M., Mulsant, B.H., Vanderbilt, J., Dodge, H.H., & Ganguli, M. (2004). Depression after stroke: A prospective epidemiological study. *Journal of American Geriatric Society, 52,* 774-778.

In: Subarachnoid Hemorrhage
Editor: Linda R. Gray

ISBN: 978-1-63463-492-2

Chapter 6

Subarachnoid Hemorrhage: Cause, Current Diagnosis and Management

***Qi Li*[1], *Gang Zhang*[1], *Sruthi Sreedharan Nambiar*[2], *Xiao Wei*[3], *Junyi Wang*[1], *Xinyue Qin*[1] *and Peng Xie*[1,*]**

[1]Department of Neurology, The First Affiliated Hospital of Chongqing Medical University, Chongqing, China

[2]Department of Medicine, Chongqing Medical University, Chongqing, China

[3]Department of Medical Technology, Chongqing Medical and Pharmaceutical College, Chongqing, China

Abstract

Subarachnoid hemorrhage (SAH) can be classified as spontaneous or traumatic bleeding into the subarachnoid space. It is usually followed by a head injury or due to aneurysmal rupture. Aneurysmal SAH is often a devastating that usually affects the younger population and is associated with high morbidity and mortality. Chronic smoking, heavy alcoholism,

* Correspondence to: Professor Peng Xie or Dr. Qi Li, Department of Neurology, The First Affiliated Hospital of Chongqing Medical University, Chongqing, China. Email: peng_xie@yahoo.com or qili_md@yahoo.com

Qi Li and Gang Zhang contributed equally to this work.

hypertension, atherosclerosis, late pregnancy are well-documented risk factors for SAH. The basic and foremost diagnostic test includes non-contrast Computed Tomography (CT) and lumbar puncture should be performed in suspected patients with negative CT scan results. Further analysis of the underlying causes of SAH should be performed by using the digital subtraction angiography (DSA), computed tomography angiography(CTA) or magnetic resonance angiography(MRA). Patient age, level of consciousness and neurologic grading on admission are important predictive factors associated with poor prognosis after SAH. Common complications of SAH include rebleeding, vasospasm, delayed cerebral ischemia, hydrocephalus.

The most important treatment option for management of acute SAH is to stop the ongoing bleeding via immediate neurosurgical or neurointerventional procedures such as clipping and coiling. A prophylactic therapy with nimodipine has shown preventive effects so as to control the rebleeding episodes in the later phase. Early identification and prompt management of SAH is crucial for improving the prognosis.

Introduction

Subarachnoid hemorrhage (SAH) can be defined as spontaneous (non-traumatic) or traumatic bleeding into the subarachnoid space. The incidence of SAH varies greatly worldwide and regionally high incidences have been reported in Finland and Japan [1]. SAH accounts for approximately 5% among all stroke subtypes with an estimated 8-10 per 100,000 per year [2]. It is usually followed by a head injury (traumatic) or due to (non-traumatic) aneurysmal rupture. Studies have revealed that it affects the younger population more often and is associated with chronic smoking, heavy alcoholism, hypertension, atherosclerosis, late pregnancy and also a minor linkage with inheritance.

Even though the clinical presentation of SAH could range from mild to extremely annihilating symptoms, '*thunderclap headache*' i.e. the sudden onset of a very severe headache; is the most common presenting symptom for SAH. Associated signs and symptoms include vomiting, visual disturbances, meningeal irritation signs and even coma. The signs and symptoms are dependent upon the location and severity of the ongoing bleeding and consequent mass effect.

The basic and foremost diagnostic test includes non-contrast computed tomography (CT) [3]. CT is highly sensitive for detection of SAH on the first day of SAH with typical distribution of bleeding in the subarachnoid space.

In highly suspected patients with negative CT scans, lumbar puncture should be performed for confirmatory diagnosis. Other tests for further analysis of the blood vessels includedigital subtraction angiogram (DSA), magnetic resonance angiography (MRA) and computed tomography angiography (CTA). DSA is the current gold standard for imaging of aneurysms and should be performed in patients if a bleeding source was not identified on CTA/MRA and the patient has a typical SAH on CT. The primary cause of highest mortality rate is the bleeding itself during the acute phase and secondary complications including rebleeding and vasospasm in the later phase.

Treatment goal for SAH is to identify the cause and stop the ongoing bleeding via immediate neurosurgical or radiological interventions such as clipping and coiling [4]. A prophylactic therapy with nimodipine has shown preventive effects so as to control the rebleeding episodes in the later phase. Although the diagnosis and management options have been improved in recent years, the prognosis of SAH still remains poor with high mortality and morbidity.

Epidemiology

SAH accounts for approximately 2-7% of all the hemorrhagic strokes. [5] The annual incidence of SAH varied greatly among different countries [6]. Geographically, Japan and Finland have been reported to have three to four folds of incidences in contrast with China having the least incidences so far when compared to other nations worldwide. [7,8] In the past years, several studies investigated the correlation of the SAH prevalence with gender, race and location.The pattern of incidences seems to increase with respect to progressing age. SAH seems to be more popular among the young aged and females than older males [9].

Etiology

SAH can be spontaneousor traumatic. Trauma is the most common cause of brain injuries.Traumatic SAH still constitutes about 4% of all cases [10]. On the basis of basic pathophysiology, the aneurysmal SAH is the most common cause of spontaneous SAH. Aneurysmal rupture comprise about 85% of all the non-traumatic or spontaneous SAH. Most of the spontaneous SAH are detectable by angiography, but 15-20% go undetected on a first angiogram [11]. About half of these concealed aneurysms are assigned to non-aneurysmal perimesencephalic subarachnoid hemorrhage (NAPSAH) and the rest to the arteriovenous malformations like moyamoya disease, cerebral amyloid angiopathy (CAA), neoplasia, bleeding disorders, etc. [1,12,13] Recent studies have been able to gradually improve the older thesis about the risk of aneurysmal rupture on the basis of its increased size since the number of small aneurysmal ruptures reported outnumbered the bigger sized aneurysms. [1,13]. The modifiable risk factors of SAH include as smoking, hypertension, and excessive alcohol abusesubject [1,13-16]. Recent studies suggest that postmenopausal state and oral contraceptives use may also contribute to a small increase of the SAH risk [16]. Several inheritable disorders including autosomal dominant polycystic kidney disease (ADPKD), Ehlers-Danlos disease IV, neurofibromatosis type 1 and Marfan's syndrome [17-19]. Adrenergics like phenylpropanolamine and cocaine abuse are also associated with both aneurysmal and nonaneurysmal SAH. [1,20,21] Several factors such as previous use of antihypertensive drugs, administration of NSAIDs , COX-2 selective inhibitors, statins withdrawal and vitamin K antagonists showed remarkable elevated incidences [22-24] . An abrupt high arterial pressure due to an intense physical exertion like strenuous exercise, sexual intercourse of any kind are evident to cause an acute onset of SAH in some patients [25-27]. Furthermore, Caucasoid race, hormone replacement therapy, hypercholesterolemia, and diabetes seem to have vague protective mechanisms. [28]

Pathophysiology

Aneurysmal rupture persists as the primary cause leading to other fatal consequences.Aneurysms seem to be more often acquired rather than congenital [1-3] .Dysfunctional hemodynamics and the fact that microscopically, cerebral arteries are deficit of inbuilt external elastic lamina and a very thin adventitia which govern most part of the explanation for the development of aneurysms. Recent studies suggest that size and location of the aneurysm have been useful for predicting the risk of rupture of an aneurysm [29]. An aneurysmal rupture episode is always followed by a cascade of destructive events from eruptive bleeding into the subarachnoid space gradually invading the entire central nervous system, thus, damaging the local tissues directly [26]. The second leading cause of spontaneous SAH isarteriovenous malformations (AVMs). Other vascular abnormalities such as cranial duralarteriovenousfistulas(DAVFs) or cavernous angiomas may also contribute to SAH.

Nonaneurysmalperimesencephalic subarachnoid hemorrhage (PMSAH) is a medical condition thatseems to have a distinct etiology and prognosis from rupture of an intracranial aneurysm [30]. The PMSAH is a relatively benign condition with good clinical outcomes [31]. Several imaging studies suggest that the radiological distribution pattern of PMSAH is relatively distinct from aneurysmal SAH and the bleeding is usually confined to the anterior aspects of the brain stem, either encircling the cisterns , concealed within the lateral Sylvian fissures or sometimes partly spreading towards the anterior interhemispheric fissures with or without affecting the ventricular system [32-34].

Most of the studies tried to link permesencephalic non-aneurysmal hemorrhage to the roots of venous origin [35].

Non-aneurysmal perimesencephalic subarachnoid hemorrhage has a less complicated pathogenesis due to the limited pattern of bleeding into the cisterns surrounding the mesencephalon.Although perimesencephalic non-aneurysmal SAH has a better clinical scenario with lower tendencies to develop complications, knowledge of the permesencephalic non-aneurysmal hemorrhage is helpful for early diagnosis and treatment.

Diagnosis

Clinical Manifestations

The clinical presentation of SAH may give a clue to the diagnosis. Patients with unrupturedintracranial aneurysms may remain asymptomatic before rupture [36]. The most characteristic symptom of subarachnoid hemorrhage is severe headache.Although a positive history of some physically exerting activities preceding the onset of the headache is not uncommon, some patients may have abrupt onset of headache at rest. A careful past history and family history may be able to consider a previous head trauma or any genetic predisposing factors respectively providing strengthening the diagnostic criteria for SAH [37,38]. A 'sentinel bleed or warning leak' must be looked upon with emphasis.Patients often complain of acute onset of severe headache defined as the "worst headache in their lifetime" which can help to provide with a primary clinical diagnosis of SAH and the patient must be examined either to confirm or to rule it out and search for the cause. Accompanying signs and symptoms include impaired consciousness levels, nausea, vomiting, nuchal rigidity, meningeal irritations signs, visual disturbances, focal neurological deficits. A significant proportion of patients may have decreased level of consciousness. Nuchal rigidity may occur as a result of inflammatory response to blooddegradation products. Although nuchal rigidity is common in patients with SAH, absence of the sign cannot rule out the diagnosis in patients with suspected SAH [39].

Cranial nerve palsy and some other focal neurological symptoms may occur when a cranial nerve is compressed or brain parenchyma is affected [40]. Third-nerve palsyis a well documented sign suggestive of the internal carotid artery or the posterior communicating artery aneurysms [41]. The vasoconstriction may occur after aneurysmal rupture, causing cerebral ischemia.

Imaging

In patients with suspected SAH, imaging examination shouldn't be delayed as SAH comprises to a wide spectrum of manifestations.A non-contrast head computed tomography (CT) is the best initial investigating tool used for diagnosing SAH with a high sensitivity rate of more than 95% within first six hours of the onset of headache, then gradually decreasing to 80-90% in the first 24 hours and negligible thereafter. [42-44] Although the noncontrastcranial CT scan is highly sensitive for identifying SAH, diagnostic lumbar puncture should be performed in suspected SAH patients with negative initial CT scans. The cerebrospinalfluid (CSF) should be carefully examined with proper technique. The pressure should be measured and CSF specimen should also be sent for culture. The presence of xanthochromia may give a clue to the diagnosis of SAH [45]. In patients with sudden onset of severe headache, anegative CT scan and CSF examination may rule out SAH in most cases and predict good prognosis [46].

MRI is the imaging method of choice especially after few days of onset of the headache due to its high sensitivity during this period of time when CT fails. Some MR sequences such as the proton-density–weighted images or fluidattenuatedinversion recovery images may provide valuable information regarding the location and time of SAH [47]. However, MRI scan is highly sensitive to motion artifact and immediate MRI scan is not available in many institutions which have limited its use in clinical practice [48]. An advantage of MRI over CT is that it provides more information about the brain and may give a clue to the diagnosis of AVM. Magnetic resonance angiography (MRA) is also an alternative imaging method for detection of intracranial aneurysms. However, the relatively low spacial resolution of MRA has limited its clinical use in the setting of SAH.

In spite of so many advantages, CT scan and MRI cannot provide essential information regarding thecause of the SAH. Angiographic studies should be performed to further elucidate the cause of SAH. Digital subtraction angiography is the gold standard for detection and characterization of intracranial aneurysms. However, it is a relatively expensive and invasive technique that was associated with risk of permanent neurologic complications [49]. Computed tomographic angiography has increasingly been used as a noninvasive screening technique for intracranial aneurysms. Recent studies suggest that the diagnostic accuracy of multidetector CT angiography is approaching that of DSA for the detection of intracranial aneurysms [50]. The introduction of recent generation CT scanners has improved the accuracy of CT angiography in neurovascular imaging. New generation spiral CT scanner offers rapid acquisition of data sets and allows reconstruction in the workstation without loss of spatial resolution. In addition to the improved data acquisition, state-of-artpostprocessing techniques may also improve the detection of aneurysms. CTA is a rapid, readily available imaging method for detection of larger aneurysms [51].

However, CT angiography has limited sensitivity for detecting aneurysms smaller than 3 mm [52]. The diagnostic accuracy of CTA for aneurysm detection is affected by many factors such as the image acquisition protocol, postprocessing technique, aneurysm size, location and the reader experience. In recent years, 3D DSA has been used as the new standard imaging method of choice for detection of intracranial aneurysms. Conventional DSA may have missed some extremely small aneurysms that could be identified on 3D DSA images. Therefore, 3D DSA should be used as the new gold standard for detection of intracranial aneurysms [53].

Treatment

General Management

SAH is a medical emergency that requires prompt diagnosis and early treatment. Emergencymedical services should be ready for the timely evaluation and transport of SAH. On admission, the neurologists should quickly performed neurological exam toidentify the level of consciousness or any existing neurological deficit [2]. Imaging studies should be performed to identify the cause of bleeding. The initial medical management of SAH is to monitor the vital signs and maintain airway. Airway surveillance is important in patients with decreased level of consciousness. Endotracheal intubation should be considered if respiratory compromise is present [3]. In comatose patients, nasogastric tube should be placed to prevent possible aspiration.Bedrest should be recommended in patients with SAH to reduce the chance ofrebleeding.

Management of Rebleeding

Ruptured cerebral aneurysms should be managed with surgical clipping or endovascular coiling to prevent rebleeding [54]. The endovascular coiling of aneurysms was described by Guglielmi in early 1990s. The detachable platinum coils was named after Guglielm and used in clinical practice [55]. The procedure includes introducing the detachable coil into the sac of the aneurysm using catheter guided bymicroguidewire. The aneurysm is occluded with the coil and the coil-induced thrombosis. The clinical application of the technique has been increasingly used worldwide and technical renovations have been made during the past 2 decades. In recent years, the coiling of aneurysms developed so fast that it has graduallyreplaced surgical occlusion as the method of choice for treatment of intracranial aneurysms. Several large randomised trialshas compared surgical clipping and endovascular coiling for treatment of intracranial aneurysms. The InternationalSubarachnoid Aneurysm Trial (ISAT) trial has enrolled 2143 patients with ruptured intracranial aneurysms and randomly classified the patients into surgical clipping or endovascular coiling. The authors found that 23.7% of patients receiving endovascular coiling were dependent or dead at 1 year follow-up as compared with 30.6% allocated neurosurgical treatment [56].

Since the outcomein patients with ruptured intracranial aneurysms is probably better with endovascular coiling than endovascular coiling, endovascular coiling are preferred method of choice in patients with aneurismal SAH. However, the outcome of SAH is predominantly determined by theseverity of SAH and the preoperativeneurological status of the patient. Therefore, both endovascularcoiling and surgical clipping are beneficial after SAH. The treatment method should be determined on an individual basis and be judged by experienced neurovascular surgeons and endovascular interventionists.

Management of Vasospasm

Vasospasm is a devastating complication after aneurysmal SAH. It is the delayed narrowing of cerebral vessels which develops 3 to 5days after the hemorrhage. The vasospasm usually reaches its peak at one to two weeks and gradually resolved after 2 to 4 weeks [57]. Transcranial Doppler (TCD) or CT angiography could be used to monitor for vasospasm [58]. Delayed ischemic deficit may occur in some patients with vasospasm and is manifested by thehemisphericfocal deficits or a reduction in thelevel of consciousness. Vasospasm contributes to a significant proportion of patient death in those who survived the initial insult. Calcium channel blockers may improve functional outcome in patients withvasospasm induced by aneurysmal subarachnoid hemorrhage. The current recommended drug is nimodipine at 60 mg taken orally every 4 h, and to be continued for 3 weeks. Hypomagnesaemia is not common in patientswith SAH and may lead to delayed ischemia. Therefore, magnesium sulphatemight be used in patients with vasospasm [2,3]. Hypervolaemia, hemodilution andhypertension treatment (Triple H therapy) has been used to treat vasospasm and delayed cerebral ischemia in the past. However, the effect of the triple H therapy is still controversial. The efficacy has not been validated in large randomizedcontrolled trials.

Management of Hydrocephalus

Hydrocephalus is a devastating neurological complication after SAH. Acute hydrocephalus may occur 24 to 72 hours after SAH and is manifested with ventricular enlargement on non-contrast enhanced CT scan [59]. Patients with acute hydrocephalus may present with obtundation and slow pupilary responses to light. Ventricular enlargement is a characteristic finding in patients with hydrocephalus. Butintraventricular hemorrhage is not always present. The presence of hydrocephalus is associated with poor functional outcome if untreated [60]. Hydrocephalus could be managed by ventriculostomy or ventriculoperitonealshunts. These surgical procedures may improve clinical outcome in patients with hydrocephalus. Now it is recommended that CSF diversion with ventriculoperitonealshunts is probably beneficial in symptomatic patients with chronic hydrocephalus [2,3].

Acknowledgments

This paper is supported by a grant from National Natural Science Foundation of China (No. 81200899).

References

[1] Feigin VL, Lawes CM, Bennett DA, Anderson CS. Stroke epidemiology: a review of population-based studies of incidence, prevalence, and case-fatality in the late 20th century. *Lancet Neurol.* 2003; 2: 43–53.

[2] Connolly ES Jr, Rabinstein AA, Carhuapoma JR, et al. Guidelines for the management of aneurismal subarachnoid hemorrhage: a guideline for healthcare professionals from the American Heart Association/American Stroke Association. *Stroke* 2012; 43: 1711–1737.

[3] Brainin M, Barnes M, Baron JC, et al. Guidance for the preparation of neurological management guidelines by EFNS scientific task forces – revised recommendations 2004. *Eur. J. Neurol.* 2004; 11: 577–581.

[4] vanGijn J, Rinkel GJ. Subarachnoid hemorrhage: diagnosis, causes and management. *Brain.* 2001; 124:249-78.

[5] G J Rinkel, J van Gijn and E F Wijdicks. Subarachnoid hemorrhage without detectable aneurysm. A review of the causes.*Stroke.*1993; 24; 1403-1409.

[6] Linn FH, Rinkel GJ, Algra A, van Gijn J. Incidence of Subarachnoid Hemorrhage Role of Region, Year, and Rate of Computed Tomography: A Meta-Analysis *Stroke.* 1996;27:625-9.

[7] Nilsson OG, Lindgren A, Ståhl N, Brandt L, Säveland H. Incidence of intracerebral and subarachnoid hemorrhage in southern Sweden. *J. Neurol.Neurosurg. Psychiatry.* 2000;69:601-7.

[8] Ingall T, Asplund K, Mähönen M, Bonita R. A Multinational Comparison of Subarachnoid Hemorrhage Epidemiology in the WHO MONICA Stroke Study Stroke. 2000;31:1054-61.

[9] deRooij NK, Linn FH, van der Plas JA, Algra A, Rinkel GJ. Incidence of subarachnoid hemorrhage: a systematic review with emphasis on region, age, gender and time trends. *J. Neurol.Neurosurg. Psychiatry.* 2007;78:1365-72.

[10] Parchani A, El-Menyar A, Al-Thani H, et al. Traumatic Subarachnoid Hemorrhage Due To Motor Vehicle Crash Versus Fall From Height: A 4-Year Epidemiological Study.*World Neurosurg*. 2014 Jun 16.

[11] Rinkel GJ, van Gijn J, Wijdicks EF. Subarachnoid Hemorrhage without Detectable Aneurysm. A review of the causes. *Stroke*. 1993 ;24:1403-9.

[12] Alcalá-Cerra GA, Moscote-Salazar LR, Barrios RS, Niño-Hernández LM, Gutiérrez Paternina. Non-aneurysmal subarachnoid hemorrhage as presentation of moyamoya disease in an adult.*J. Surg. Neurol. Int.* 2011;2:80.

[13] Van Gijn J, Kerr RS, Rinkel GJ. Subarachnoid hemorrhage. *Lancet* 2007;369:306-18.

[14] Qureshi AI, Suarez JI, Parekh PD, Sung G, Geocadin R, Bhardwaj A, Tamargo RJ, Ulatowski JA. Risk factors for multiple intracranial aneurysms.*Neurosurgery*. 1998;43:22-6.

[15] Qureshi AI, Sung GY, Suri MF, Straw RN, Guterman LR, Hopkins LN.Factors associated with aneurysm size in patients with subarachnoid hemorrhage: effect of smoking and aneurysm location.*Neurosurgery*. 2000;46:44-50.

[16] Mhurchu CN, Anderson C, Jamrozik K, et al. Hormonal factors and risk of aneurysmal subarachnoid hemorrhage: an international population-based, case-control study. *Stroke* 2001; 32:606.

[17] Soejima M, Sugita Y, Koda Y. An autopsy case of subarachnoid hemorrhage due to ruptured cerebral aneurysm associated with polycystic kidney disease caused by a novel PKD1 mutation. *Forensic Sci Int.* 2014 Jul 2. pii: S0379-0738(14)00265-5.

[18] Vlak MH1, Algra A, Brandenburg R, Rinkel GJ. Prevalence of unruptured intracranial aneurysms, with emphasis on sex, age, comorbidity, country, and time period: a systematic review and meta-analysis. *Lancet Neurol*. 2011;10:626-36.

[19] Hussain I, Duffis EJ, Gandhi CD, Prestigiacomo CJ. Genome-wide association studies of intracranial aneurysms: an update. *Stroke*. 2013;44:2670-5.

[20] Kernan WN, Viscoli CM, Brass LM, et al. Phenylpropanolamine and the risk of hemorrhagic stroke. *N. Engl. J. Med.* 2000; 343:1826.

[21] Yoon BW, Bae HJ, Hong KS, et al. Phenylpropanolamine contained in cold remedies and risk of hemorrhagic stroke. *Neurology* 2007; 68:146.

[22] Risselada R, Straatman H, van Kooten F, et al. Withdrawal of statins and risk of subarachnoid hemorrhage.*Stroke* 2009; 40:2887.

[23] Garbe E1, Kreisel SH, Behr S. Risk of subarachnoid hemorrhage and early case fatality associated with outpatient antithrombotic drug use..*Stroke.* 2013;44:2422-6.

[24] Risselada R, Straatman H, van Kooten F, et al. Platelet aggregation Inhibitors, vitamin K antagonists and risk of subarachnoid hemorrhage.*J.Thromb.Haemost.* 2011;9:517-23.

[25] Vlak MH1, Rinkel GJ, Greebe P, van der Bom JG, AlgraA. Trigger factors and their attributable risk for rupture of intracranial aneurysms: a case- crossover study. *Stroke.* 2011;42:1878-82.

[26] Anderson C, Ni Mhurchu C, Scott D, Bennett D, Jamrozik K, Hankey G. Triggers of subarachnoid hemorrhage: role of physical exertion, smoking, and alcohol in the AustralasianCooperative Research on Subarachnoidhemorrhage Study (ACROSS); Australasian Cooperative Research on Subarachnoid Hemorrhage Study Group. *Stroke.* 2003;34:1771-6.

[27] Alawi A, Mehta S, Edgell R. Post-coital MCA Dissection Presenting with SAH: A Case Report and Review of the Literature. *J.Neurointerv.Surg.* 2014;6Suppl 1:A72-3.

[28] Feigin VL, Rinkel GJ, Lawes CM, Algra A, Bennett DA, van Gijn J, Anderson CS. Risk factors for subarachnoid hemorrhage: an updated systematic review of epidemiological studies.*Stroke.* 2005;36:2773-80.

[29] Kashiwazaki D, Kuroda S; Sapporo SAH Study Group.Size ratio can highly predict rupture risk in intracranial small (<5 mm) aneurysms Sapporo SAH Study Group. *Stroke.* 2013;44:2169-73.

[30] Anderson RC, Baskin J, Feldstein NA. Perimesencephalicnonaneurysmal subarachnoid hemorrhage in the pediatric population: Case report and review of the literature. *Pediatr.Neurosurg.* 2002;37:258–261.

[31] vanGijn J, van Dongen KJ, Vermeulen M, et al. Perimesencephalic hemorrhage: A nonaneurysmal and benign form of subarachnoid hemorrhage. *Neurology.* 1985;35:493–497.

[32] Schievink WI, Wijdicks EFM. Pretruncal subarachnoid hemorrhage: An anatomically correct description of the perimesencephalic subarachnoid hemorrhage. *Stroke.* 1997;28:2572.

[33] Schwartz TH, Mayer SA. Quadrigeminal variant of perimesencephalicnonaneurysmal subarachnoid hemorrhage. *Neurosurgery*. 2000;46:584–588.

[34] Marder CP, Narla V, Fink JR, Tozer Fink KR. Subarachnoid hemorrhage: beyond aneurysms. *AJR Am. J.Roentgenol.* 2014;202:25-37.

[35] van der Schaaf IC, Velthuis BK, Gouw A, et al. Venous drainage in perimesencephalic hemorrhage. *Stroke*. 2004;35:1614–1618.

[36] Bassi P, Bandera R, Loiero M, Tognoni G, Mangoni A. Warning signs in subarachnoid hemorrhage: a cooperative study. *Acta Neurol. Scand.* 1991;84:277–281.

[37] Schievink WI. Intracranial aneurysms. *N. Engl. J. Med.* 1997;336:28–40.

[38] Fontanarosa PB. Recognition of subarachnoid hemorrhage. *Ann.Emerg.Med.* 1989;18:1199 –1205.

[39] Mayberg MR. Warning leaks and subarachnoid hemorrhage. *West J Med.* 1990;153:549 –550.

[40] Edlow JA. Diagnosis of subarachnoid hemorrhage in the emergency department. *Emerg. Med.Clin. North Am.* 2003;21:73– 87.

[41] Edlow JA. Diagnosis of subarachnoid hemorrhage. *Neurocrit Care.* 2005;2:99 –109.

[42] Sames TA, Storrow AB, Finkelstein JA, Magoon MR. Sensitivity of new-generation computed tomography in subarachnoid hemorrhage. *AcadEmerg Med.* 1996;3:16 –20.

[43] Tomasello F, d'Avella D, de Divitiis O. Does lamina terminalis fenestration reduce the incidence of chronic hydrocephalus after subarachnoid hemorrhage? *Neurosurgery.* 1999;45:827– 831.

[44] van der Wee N, Rinkel GJ, Hasan D, van Gijn J. Detection of subarachnoid hemorrhage on early CT: is lumbar puncture still needed after a negative scan? *J. Neurol.Neurosurg. Psychiatry.* 1995;58:357–359.

[45] Sidman R, Connolly E, Lemke T. Subarachnoid hemorrhage diagnosis: lumbar puncture is still needed when the computed tomography scan is normal. *AcadEmerg. Med.* 1996;3:827– 831.

[46] vanGijn J, van Dongen KJ. The time course of aneurysmal haemorrhage on computed tomograms. *Neuroradiology.* 1982;23:153–156.

[47] Mitchell P, Wilkinson ID, Hoggard N, et al. Detection of subarachnoid hemorrhage with magnetic resonance imaging. *J. Neurol.Neurosurg. Psychiatry.* 2001;70:205–211.

[48] Yuan MK, Lai PH, Chen JY, et al. Detection of subarachnoid hemorrhage at acute and subacute/chronic stages: comparison of four magnetic resonance imaging pulse sequences and computed tomography. *J. Chin. Med. Assoc.* 2005;68:131–137.

[49] Cloft HJ, Joseph GJ, Dion JE. Risk of cerebral angiography in patients with subarachnoid hemorrhage, cerebral aneurysm, and arteriovenous malformation: a meta-analysis. *Stroke* 1999;30(2):317–320.

[50] Wintermark M, Uske A, Chalaron M, et al. Multislice computerized tomography angiography in the evaluation of intracranial aneurysms: a comparison with intraarterial digital subtraction angiography. *J.Neurosurg.*2003;98(4):828–836.

[51] White PM, Wardlaw JM, Easton V. Can noninvasive imaging accurately depict intracranial aneurysms? a systematic review. *Radiology* 2000;217(2):361–370.

[52] Sakamoto S, Kiura Y, Shibukawa M, Ohba S, Arita K, Kurisu K. Subtracted 3D CT angiography for evaluation of internal carotid artery aneurysms: comparison with conventional digital subtraction angiography. *AJNR Am. J. Neuroradiol.*2006;27(6):1332–1337.

[53] McKinney AM, Palmer CS, Truwit CL, Karagulle A, Teksam M. Detection of aneurysms by 64-section multidetector CT angiography in patients acutely suspected of having an intracranial aneurysm and comparison with digital subtraction and 3D rotational angiography. *AJNR Am. J. Neuroradiol.*2008;29(3):594–602.

[54] Van der Schaaf IC, Algra A, Wermer MJH, et al. Endovascular coiling versus neurosurgical clipping for patients with aneurismal subarachnoid hemorrhage. *Cochrane Database Syst. Rev.*2005;4: CD003085.

[55] Guglielmi G, Vinuela F, Dion J, Duckwiler G. Electrothrombosis of saccular aneurysms via endovascular approach, part 2: preliminary clinical experience. *J.Neurosurg.* 1991;75:8 –14.

[56] Molyneux A, Kerr R, Stratton I, et al. International Subarachnoid Aneurysm Trial (ISAT) of neurosurgical clipping versus endovascular coiling in 2143 patients with ruptured intracranial aneurysms: a randomised trial. *Lancet* 2002; 360: 1267–74.

[57] Kassell NF, Boarini DJ, Adams HP Jr, et al. Overall management of ruptured aneurysm: comparison ofearly and late operation. *Neurosurgery.* 1981;9:120 –128.

[58] Klingelhofer J, Dander D, Holzgraefe M, Bischoff C, Conrad B.Cerebral vasospasm evaluated by transcranial Doppler ultrasonography at different intracranial pressures. *J.Neurosurg.* 1991;75:752–758.

[59] Black PM. Hydrocephalus and vasospasm after subarachnoid hemorrhagefrom ruptured intracranial aneurysms. *Neurosurgery.* 1986;18:12–16.
[60] vanGijn J, Hijdra A, Wijdicks EF, Vermeulen M, van Crevel H. Acutehydrocephalus after aneurysmal subarachnoid hemorrhage. *J.Neurosurg.*1985;63:355–362.

In: Subarachnoid Hemorrhage
Editor: Linda R. Gray

ISBN: 978-1-63463-492-2

Chapter 7

Decompressive Craniectomy for Management of Intracranial Hypertension in Poor-Grade Aneurysmal Subarachnoid Hemorrhage

Naoki Otani*[*], *Yoshio Takasato and Kentaro Mori
Department of Neurosurgery, National Defense Medical College, Tokorozawa, Saitama, Japan

Abstract

Patients with poor-grade aneurysmal subarachnoid hemorrhage (SAH) frequently suffer devastating sequelae caused by the primary and secondary impacts on the brain, particularly if associated with large intracerebral hematoma, sylvian hematoma, or acute subdural hematoma, which result in poor outcomes due to the significant brain stem compression caused by the mass effect. The optimum treatment for aneurysmal SAH is early surgical intervention to prevent re-bleeding and for safer management of vasospasm after aneurysm obliteration.

[*] Corresponding author: Naoki Otani, M.D., Department of Neurosurgery, National Defense Medical College, 3-2 Namiki, Tokorozawa, Saitama 359-8513, Japan, Tel: +81-4-2995-1656; Fax: +81-4-2996-5207; e-mail: naotani@ndmc.ac.jp.

However, severe malignant vasospasm caused by SAH may develop and become resistant to conventional medical and endovascular treatments, resulting in extensive infarction and edema with secondary increased intracranial pressure (ICP) and decreased brain blood perfusion. Decompressive craniectomy (DC) is known to reduce the morbidity and mortality in critically ill patients with massive ischemic infarction and severe head injury. However, the role of DC in the treatment of SAH patients is not fully understood. Several experimental studies have indicated that DC significantly improves functional outcome due to decreased ICP or increasced perfusion pressure. Clinical reports about the efficacy of DC for the treatment of poor-grade aneurysmal SAH are reviewed and discussed here.

Keywords: Brain stem compression, massive ischemic infarction, subarachnoid hemorrhage, cerebral angiography, intracranial hypertension

Introduction

Poor-grade aneurysmal subarachnoid hemorrhage (SAH) has both primary and secondary impacts on the brain frequently resulting in devastating outcome, particularly if associated with the formation of large intracerebral hematoma (ICH), sylvian hematoma, or acute subdural hematoma (ASDH), the mass effect of which cause significant brain stem compression. Decompressive craniectomy (DC) is known to reduce the morbidity and mortality in critically ill patients with massive ischemic infarction [13, 30, 37, 53] and severe head injury [1, 43]. However, the effects of DC in the treatment of poor-grade SAH remain obscure. Recent studies suggested that DC with dural plasty intended to enlarge the intracranial space allows the swollen cerebral hemisphere to expand out of the normal cranial limits, thus avoiding progression of brain herniation, which results in improvement of cerebral compliance and decreased intracranial pressure (ICP), and improves in both cerebral blood flow and cerebral microvascular perfusion, possibly accompanied by higher levels of brain tissue oxygen [9, 10, 32]. Therefore, DC might be an effective strategy for the treatment of poor-grade SAH [15, 56, 57]. The present study reviewed experimental and clinical reports describing the efficacy of DC for patients with poor-grade aneurysmal SAH.

Surgical Management

Aggressive resuscitation such as tracheal intubation and adequate ventilation under sedation was performed in the emergency room. The diagnosis of SAH was confirmed by computed tomography (CT). To prevent aneurysmal rebleeding during the acute stage, the systolic blood pressure was actively lowered to <120 mmHg. All patients immediately underwent cerebral angiography after stabilization. During surgery, osmotic diuresis (mannitol 1-2 mg/kg) and cerebrospinal fluid (CSF) drainage were performed if necessary to slacken the brain.

Surgical Procedure

Primary DC and standard microscopic techniques were usually performed to obliterate the aneurysm. Standard treatment for ruptured aneurysms in our clinic is clipping the neck of the aneurysm within the first 24 hours. An intraventricular CSF drainage catheter was routinely inserted in patients with World Federation of Neurosurgical Societies (WFNS) score of 3 or more, and in some patients with WFNS score of 2 or less according to the surgeon's personal assessment of complication risk. The surgical procedure was as follows. A generous craniotomy flap was removed via a large reversed question mark scalp incision with the following margins: anteriorly, frontal to the floor of the anterior cranial fossa; superiorly, within 2 cm of the superior sagittal sinus; posteriorly, within 1 cm of the asterion; and inferiorly, to the floor of the middle fossa (Figure 1A-D). The dura was opened with a semicircular incision with additional dural incisions for decompression. Intraoperative hyperventilation was not routinely performed, and intraoperative hypotension was avoided to maintain appropriate perfusion pressure. The aneurysm was clipped and the hematoma was evacuated.

Postoperative Management

Patients were aggressively treated postoperatively to avoid intracranial hypertension and vasospasm with ICP monitoring in the neurological intensive care unit. The ICP was continuously monitored in all patients using a subdural fiber optic ICP catheter (Camino Laboratories, San Diego, CA, USA) for at least one week. If ICP remained at >20 mmHg after medical treatment, mild hypothermia therapy was induced by surface cooling and continued for 3 days with the target temperature of 35°C in principle. In addition, CSF was drained to decrease the ICP caused by hydrocephalus. To prevent cerebral vasospasm, prophylactic normovolemic~hypervolemic hyperdynamic therapy was continued for at least 2 weeks after surgery including intravenous administration of calcium channel antagonists and plasma volume expansion through the infusion of albumin and/or low molecular weight dextran to maintain the serum colloid oncotic pressure. Patients developing new neurologic deficit (decreased consciousness, hemiparesis, aphasia) or suspicious systemic signs (headache, unexplained fever) in the postoperative period, especially day 4~14 after ictus, immediately underwent brain CT. Patients with radiologic ischemic signs corresponding to the vascular territory were diagnosed with cerebral vasospasm. Patients with normal radiologic findings without ischemic changes immediately underwent digital subtraction angiography to confirm the diagnosis. With this approach, early diagnosis of vasospasm could be established before deterioration of the patient's condition due to late complications of edema and herniation, and treatment was started immediately after the diagnosis was made. Nicardipine hydrochloride, a calcium channel blocker, was also used in our department in the standard treatment of cerebral vasospasm. Patients not responding to hypertensive-hypervolemic-hemodilution therapy were managed with balloon angioplasty in the time period of 6–12 hours from the onset of the symptoms. The cranial bone flap was replaced 1–2 months after the initial surgery.

Representative Case and Case Series

A 57-year-old man suffered sudden onset of headache with loss of consciousness. CT on admission showed diffuse SAH with ICH (Figure 2A, 2B). Three-dimensional CT angiography revealed a large aneurysm at the internal carotid artery bifurcation. The patient underwent aneurysm clipping with primary DC (Figure 2E). Two days after the operation, the brain edema had progressively worsened, but the midline shift and brain stem compression had improved (Figure 2C, 2D). The patient recovered with Glasgow Outcome Scale score of moderate disability.

In addition, 141 consecutive patients with poor-grade SAH (grades IV and V) were treated in our hospital. We retrospectively reviewed the hospital records including medical charts, operative records, and radiological findings

(Table 1). Patient outcome was assessed on discharge using the Glasgow Outcome Scale of five levels: good recovery, moderate disability, severe disability, vegetative state, and death. We divided the clinical outcomes of the patients into four groups with or without DC and in grade IV or V, which showed that favorable outcome increased after DC (Figure 3).

Discussion

Surgical Outcome in Poor-Grade Aneurysmal SAH Patients

Aneurysmal SAH is associated with significant morbidity and mortality [68]. Initial clinical grades IV and V as well as initial Fisher grades III and IV are strongly associated with poor outcome [50]. In addition, the presence of intracerebral or intraventricular hemorrhage has been identified as one of the common factors affecting the outcome [47, 48]. Early aggressive surgery and intensive care for SAH patients in poor clinical condition can improve the mortality and morbidity [4, 11, 33, 55]. Previously, increased ICP has been associated with poor-grade aneurysmal SAH [4], with dismal outcome irrespective of aggressive management. Surgical outcome continues to be unfavorable in many patients with poor-grade SAH despite recent advances in treatment because of uncontrollable intracranial hypertension. Further advances in cerebral aneurysm treatment and neurointensive care have attained favorable outcome in half of poor-grade SAH patients if ICP could be controlled to reduce secondary brain injury [34, 69]. Increased ICP is associated with several detrimental effects such as cerebral ischemia following reduced perfusion pressure [20]. Intractable intracranial hypertension is associated with poor outcome in patients with poor-grade aneurysmal SAH [27, 34, 35, 63]. Therefore, immediate and continued effective ICP management is associated with improved outcome [4].

Pathophysiology of Poor-Grade SAH with Hematoma

The clinical outcome for SAH patients with ICH is usually worse than that for SAH patients without ICH [4, 5, 19]. ICP increased in over half of all patients with SAH, particularly among those with poor-grade SAH and ICH [21]. On the other hand, the clinical outcome for SAH patients with ICH does not significantly differ from that of SAH patients without associated hematoma [2]. The incidence of rebleeding in patients with poor-grade SAH is 22% with ICH and 14% without ICH. Clinical grades on admission were significantly higher and outcome at 6 months after onset was less favorable in patients with poor-grade SAH with ICH than in those without ICH. Larger ICH was associated with worse clinical grade and less favorable outcome. The sites of the hematoma and ruptured aneurysm were closely correlated. The poor outcome of patients with ICH seems to be related to the severity of clinical grade on admission. However, the two groups did not significantly differ in terms of management and surgical outcome for the same clinical grades [65]. Initial brain damage caused by ICH and subsequent brain edema seemed to be the main cause of disability, and might be related to the poor clinical outcome. Intracranial hypertension in patients with SAH can be associated with deleterious changes, which might have profound impacts on outcome [72]. Consequently, aggressive clot evacuation and aneurysm obliteration are recommended.

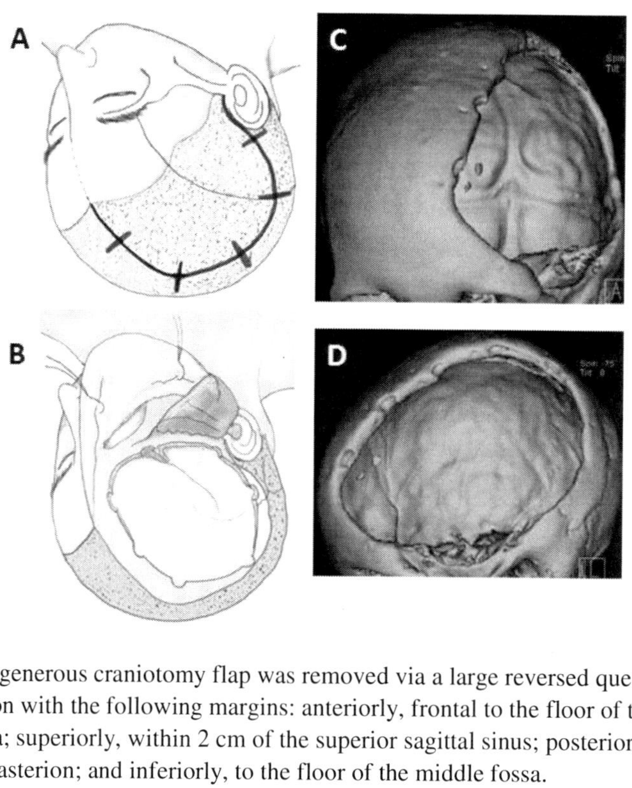

Figure 1. A generous craniotomy flap was removed via a large reversed question mark scalp incision with the following margins: anteriorly, frontal to the floor of the anterior cranial fossa; superiorly, within 2 cm of the superior sagittal sinus; posteriorly, within 1 cm of the asterion; and inferiorly, to the floor of the middle fossa.

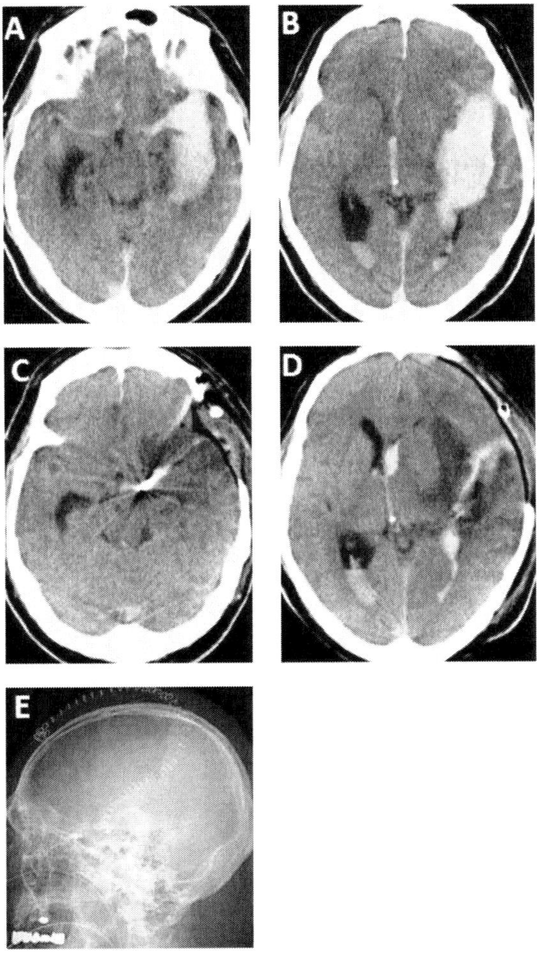

Figure 2. A 57-year-old man suffered sudden onset of headache with loss of consciousness. CT scans on admission (A, B) showing diffuse subarachnoid hemorrhage with intracerebral hematoma. Three-dimensional CT angiogram revealing a large aneurysm at the internal carotid artery bifurcation. The patient underwent aneurysm clipping with primary decompressive craniectomy (E). Two days after the operation, the brain edema had progressively worsened, but midline shift and brain stem compression improved (C, D). The patient recovered with Glasgow Outcome Scale score of moderate disability.

Intracranial hypertension after SAH can be caused by cerebral edema, intracranial hematoma, hydrocephalus, intraventricular hemorrhage, early brain injury, aneurysm rerupture, aneurysm treatment, or delayed cerebral ischemia [21]. Study of the effect of intracranial hypertension after SAH with cerebral microdialysis found that cerebral metabolic levels were severely disturbed in patients with SAH and intracranial hypertension compared to patients with normal ICP [39]. The levels of excitotoxic glutamate and membrane-degradation marker glycerol in cerebral dialysate further deteriorated 5 days after ictus, possibly reflecting secondary brain damage. ICP of more than 20 mmHg was a strong predictor of death and was associated with unfavorable neurological outcome. Cerebral infarct may develop following vasospasm or after microsurgical clipping of ruptured aneurysms, and could cause increased ICP. On the other hand, cerebral vasospasm usually peaks 4–10 days after initial hemorrhage, and can lead to delayed global cerebral edema in 20% of patients and subsequent higher ICP [14, 23]. The resulting high ICP leads to insufficient cerebral perfusion pressure, which contributes significantly to morbidity and mortality in patients with SAH [32]. Delayed cerebral infarction can also lead to similar disastrous results [52].

Rapid control of ICP has been associated with improved outcome, indicating that early control of ICP and cerebral blood flow is important to improve outcome or to prevent further deterioration. The main issue is to correct increased ICP to prevent brain herniation, so reducing ICP levels < 20 mmHg was beneficial and DC becomes an option after the failure of other methods. Several studies showed that successful management of increased ICP with less invasive approaches is efficacious and improves outcome after aneurysmal SAH and its related complications, such as edema, infarction, and/or hematoma. Consequently, refractory high ICP >20 mmHg was considered to be the main indication for DC after aneurysmal SAH [17, 38]. The management of SAH patients depends on the prevention of secondary brain damage. High ICP within the fixed volume of the skull can lead to secondary brain damage, herniation, and permanent neurological damage, or even death. High ICP in SAH patients is associated with poor outcome [58, 72]. Refractory high ICP is associated with unfavorable neurological outcome in SAH patients, but better understanding and more aggressive approaches to treat increased ICP may improve prognosis [21, 49]. Severe malignant vasospasm may also develop and become resistant to conventional medical treatment in some patients. For these reasons, new additional therapeutic strategies such as DC are essential to improve the clinical outcome in patients with poor-grade SAH. In our series, ICP of more than 20 mmHg during 7 days after ictus was a strong predictor of death and was associated with unfavorable outcome (Figure. 4). These data also suggested that early control of ICP is important to improve outcome or to prevent further deterioration.

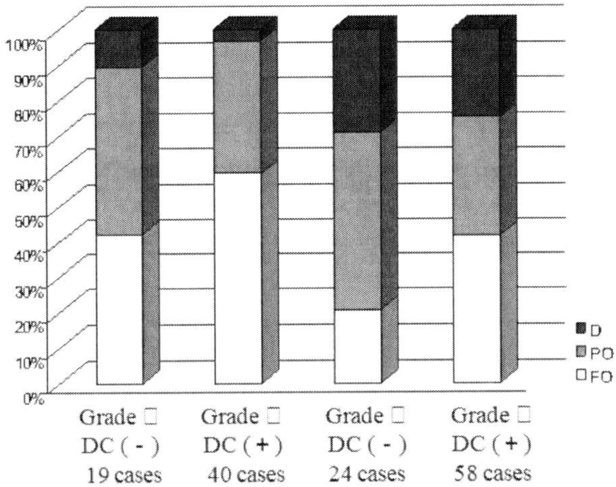

Figure 3. Clinical outcomes in our hospital for poor-grade SAH patients (grades IV and V) divided into four groups with or without DC, showing that favorable outcome increased after DC. D: death, PO: poor outcome, FO: favorable outcome.

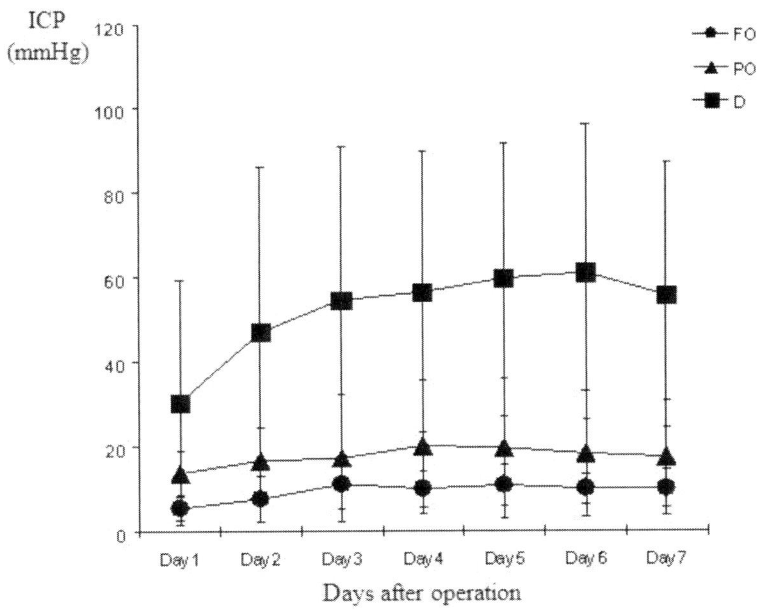

Figure 4. Time course of changes in ICP during the 7 days after surgery. ICP of all patients with favorable outcome was continuously <25 mmHg, and of those who died was continuously >25 mmHg. D: death, FO: favorable outcome, PO: poor outcome.

Table 1. Clinical characteristics of 141 patients treated for poor-grade SAH

	Grade IV		Grade V	
	DC (-)	DC (+)	DC (-)	DC (+)
Number of patients	19	40	24	58
Age (yrs)				
Range	37-77	35-72	35-75	30-74
Mean	59.4	57.2	57.8	57.1
Sex				
Male	5	17	14	24
Female	14	23	10	34
Side				
Right	11	22	12	22
Left	8	18	12	36
Aneurysm size				
Small	17	34	20	50
Medium	2	4	2	5
Large	0	2	2	3
Re-rupture	1	5	3	7
Intraoperative rupture	1	5	3	5
Hypothermia therapy	0	4	2	12
Aneurysm site				
ICA	4	11	5	18
MCA	13	27	10	37
AcomA	2	2	9	3
Hematoma volume (mm^3)	38.8	40.1	39.3	42.2
Midline shift (mm)	4.33	7.95	6.28	8.8
Basal cistern effacement				
Yes	2	6	2	5
No	17	34	22	53
Brain swelling	3	15	16	36

DC: decompressive craniectomy, ICA: internal carotid artery, MCA: middle cerebral artery, AcomA: anterior communicating artery.

Efficacy and Pathophysiology of DC

Standard therapies for treating high ICP in SAH patients are frequently adopted from experiences with treating traumatic brain injury, including optimizing cerebral venous outflow, controlled hyperventilation, CSF diversion, and surgical removal of space-occupying intracranial hematoma [45, 62]. DC is a neurosurgical procedure which is intended to treat high ICP. DC includes removal of the calvarial bones to create free space for brain expansion under the scalp, and is intended to minimize ischemic damage by increasing cerebral blood flow [3, 25, 28, 67]. Recent clinical findings suggest that external decompression might reduce ICP [22, 24, 46, 59]. Craniectomy and enlarged dural plasty induce significant decrease in ICP and increase in cerebral tissue oxygenation [24, 46]. External decompression may also significantly increase cerebral tissue oxygenation [22, 59]. In addition, clinical studies have suggested that DC results in significant elevation of mean cerebral blood flow velocity and significant decreases in the middle cerebral artery (MCA) pulsatility index, indicating reduction in cerebrovascular resistance in most patients with traumatic brain swelling [5, 8]. Recent studies have suggested that DC with dural augmentation enlarges the intracranial space so that the swollen cerebral hemisphere can expand out of the normal cranial limits, thus avoiding progression of brain herniation. Such gain in intracranial volume results in both improvement of cerebral compliance and decrease in ICP; and the latter favors increases in both cerebral blood flow and cerebral microvascular perfusion, possibly accompanied by higher brain tissue oxygen tension as well as normalization of abnormal metabolic parameters in patients with cerebral ischemia [9, 10, 32]. Therefore, DC can induce immediate reduction in ICP and control the increase in ICP that occurs several days after SAH. Surgical outcome improves in patients with ICP controlled by DC, compared with patients with uncontrolled ICP [2, 21]. In particular, delayed swelling can induce high ICP, which can be confused with the symptoms of vasospasm. Therefore, early DC would be useful to avoid this clinical problem.

Surgical Outcome of DC for SAH

Intracranial hypertension can be occurred following aneurysmal SAH. DC for SAH can be performed as primary prophylaxis as well as secondary salvage. Prophylactic DC is not intended to control refractory high ICP, but to avoid expected postsurgical increase in ICP. DC was effective to improve clinical outcome in two patients with SAH caused by ruptured anterior communicating artery aneurysm treated by bifrontal craniectomy [54] and by basilar top aneurysm treated by posterior fossa decompression [31]. DC for intractable high ICP resulted in improved cerebral tissue oxygenation in SAH patient with diffuse cerebral edema [22, 59]. DC can be performed for SAH with the aim of reducing intracranial pressure, increasing cerebral perfusion, which results in reducing further morbidity and mortality.

Recent clinical studies have found that DC can improve the surgical outcome of patients with poor-grade SAH and massive ICH [15, 56, 57]. The surgical outcome was improved by ICP control in a series of 8 patients with poor-grade MCA aneurysmal SAH and sylvian hematoma treated with external decompression, resulting in favorable outcome in 5 patients and poor outcome in 3 patients [57] Five of the eight patients enjoyed excellent or good outcome at 1 year, suggesting the potential beneficial effect of rapid control of ICP may translate into good outcome. External decompression resulted in favorable outcome rates of 33% in grade IV and 40% in grade V patients with sylvian hematoma [56]. DC led to significant decrease of medically refractory high ICP even in SAH patients without large intracranial hematoma [51]. Long-term outcome was better for patients who underwent secondary DC within the first 48 hours after SAH.

DC can be a life-saving procedure which provides better outcome in patients with cerebral infarction secondary to vasospasm and SAH [66]. DC was most beneficial if performed immediately after the detection of persistent increase in ICP in patients younger than 60 years old, suggesting that early intervention may have large effect on the outcome [66]. In general, DC for the treatment of malignant vasospasm after SAH had a favorable effect on the prognosis, but this group still had the lowest beneficial outcome compared to other groups (hematoma, stoke, trauma, etc.), ranging from 10% to 26.6% [17]. Although DC has prolonged the short-term survival of patients with poor-grade SAH and ICH, the overall quality of life experienced by survivors remains poor [15]. Further investigation is required to clarify long-term outcomes with particular focus on higher cerebral function.

DC for SAH with ASDH

The incidence of aneurysmal SAH associated with ASDH is between 0.5% and 7.9% [5, 6] and leads to poor clinical outcome [26, 71]. SAH patients with ASDH have poorer prognosis compared to SAH patients without ASDH [40]. The poor outcome in SAH patients with ASDH seems to be related to the severity of the clinical grade on admission. Initial brain damage caused by ASDH, and the subsequent brain edema, seem to be the main causes of disability, which is closely related to the poor clinical outcome. Therefore, aggressive clot evacuation and aneurysm obliteration are recommended for rapid control of the ICP, which is associated with improved outcome. Early control of the ICP and cerebral blood flow is important for improving the outcome and to prevent deterioration. In general, patients with aneurysmal SAH and ASDH tend to have worse prognosis compared to SAH patients without ASDH [27]. If patients with aneurysmal ASDH suffer no primary damage to the brain tissue, the prognosis seems to be more favorable if adequate diagnostic investigations and prompt aggressive treatment are performed. The poor outcome in patients with ASDH is probably due to the initial elevated ICP caused by the ASDH. Despite recent advances in the treatment of patients with poor-grade SAH, surgical outcome remains generally poor because of the uncontrolled intracranial hypertension. Elevated ICP has been associated with several detrimental effects, such as cerebral ischemia and reduction of the cerebral blood flow [27]. In previous series, the mortality rate was 21% and the poor outcome rate was 42% in patients with aneurysmal SAH and ASDH [29]. Favorable outcome was achieved in 41.7% of SAH patients with ASDH who underwent primary DC [42]. Therefore, rapid DC will be useful for controlling the ICP, thus improving the outcome and decreasing the mortality rates in such patients.

DC for SAH with Massive Hematoma

Recent clinical studies have reported that DC can be useful to improve the surgical outcome in patients with poor-grade SAH and massive ICH [15, 22, 46, 56]. Surgical outcome was improved by ICP control in a small series of 8 patients with poor-grade MCA aneurysmal SAH and sylvian hematoma treated with external decompression [57]. Favorable outcome was achieved in 5 of the 8 patients and poor outcome in 3 patients. Favorable outcome rates were 33% in grade V patients and 40% in grade IV patients with sylvian hematoma treated with external decompression [56]. Similarly, favorable outcome was obtained in 56.0% of grade IV patients after treatment which included decompression [41]. The ICP remained below 20 mmHg for 7 days after surgery in all patients with favorable outcome, but tended to remain at or over

20 mmHg after surgery in the patients with poor outcome. Prophylactic DC leads to favorable outcome in more than half of patients presenting with WFNS grade IV together with large ICH or sylvian hematoma. In addition, the ICP remained over 25 mmHg in the patients who died. Favorable outcomes were found in 52.6% of patients after 12 months [12]. Secondary DC resulted in favorable outcome in 72.7% of patients without infarct, but only 16.7% of patients with delayed infarct and refractory intracranial hypertension. Similarly, good outcome was obtained in 37.5% of patients without rebleeding or infarction compared to overall 26.6% among all patients treated with craniectomy after 6 months [18]. These findings suggested that patients with progressive cerebral edema may benefit most from secondary DC after SAH. DC prolonged the short-term survival of patients with poor-grade SAH with ICH, but the overall quality of life for survivors was still poor. We suggest that DC helps to reduce morbidity and mortality through control of elevated ICP in patients with poor-grade SAH associated with ICH. However, further investigation is required to clarify the value of DC for treating poor-grade SAH from the viewpoint of long-term higher cerebral function.

Complications of DC

Complications of DC can include infection, development of subdural hygroma, and sinking syndrome in the later phase of recovery, characterized by new cognitive, neurological, or psychological deficits [7, 36, 60, 61]. The development of hydrocephalus as a result of DC may be a common occurrence [44], but only a few studies have examined the association between hydrocephalus and DC for stroke [44, 70]. DC may be associated with postoperative hydrocephalus, possibly because the CSF dynamic was disturbed after part of the skull vault was removed [43, 70]. Hydrocephalus occurred in 3 (60%) of 5 patients who underwent DC for ICH followed by cranioplasty [44]. Furthermore, a short distance between the decompressive defect and the sagittal midline was associated with the development of hydrocephalus after DC in traumatic brain injury patients [16]. Investigation of the risk factors for hydrocephalus in 28 patients who underwent DC for malignant hemispheric cerebral infarction showed that DC with the superior limit <25 mm from the sagittal midline had significantly increased risk for both pre- and post-cranioplasty hydrocephalus ($p = 0.008$ and $p = 0.010$, respectively) [64]. Therefore, DC with a superior limit <25 mm from the sagittal midline should be avoided to prevent the development of hydrocephalus.

References

[1] Aarabi, B., Hesdorffer, D. C., Ahn, E. S., Aresco, C., Acalea, T. M. & Eisenberg, H. M. (2006). Outcome following decompressive craniectomy for malignant swelling due to severe head injury. *J Neurosurg*, *104*, 469-479.

[2] Abbed, K. M. & Ogilvy, C. S. (2003). Intracerebral hematoma from aneurysm rupture. *Neurosurg Focus*, *15(4)*, E4.

[3] Akyuz, M., Ucar, T., Acikbas, C., Kazan, S., Yilmaz, M. & Tuncer, R. (2010). Effect of early bilateral decompressive craniectomy on outcome for severe traumatic brain injury. *Turk Neurosurg*, *20*, 382-389.

[4] Bailes, J. E., Spetzler, R. F., Hadley, M. N., Balwin, H. Z. & Baldwin, H. Z. (1990). Management morbidity and mortality of poor grade aneurysm patients. *J Neurosurg*, *72*, 559-566.

[5] Barton, E. & Tudor, J. (1982). Subdural haematoma in association with intracranial aneurysm. *Neuroradiology*, *23*, 157-160.

[6] Bassette, C. R. & Lemmen, L. F. (1952). Subdural hematoma associated with bleeding intracranial aneurysm. *J Neurosurg*, *9*, 443-450.

[7] Bijlenga, P., Zumofen, D., Yilmaz, H., Creisson, E. & de Tribolet, N. (2007). Orthostatic mesodiencephalic dysfunction after decompressive craniectomy. *J Neurol Neurosurg Psychiatry*, *78*, 430–433.

[8] Bor-Seng-Shu, E., Hirsch, R., Teixeira, M. J., De Andrade, A. F., Marino, R. Jr. (2006). Cerebral hemodynamic changes gauged by transcranial Doppler ultrasonography in patients with posttraumatic brain swelling treated by surgical decompression. *J Neurosurg*, *104*, 93-100.

[9] Bor-Seng-Shu, E., Figueiredo, E. G., Amorim, R. L., Teixeira, M. J., Valbuza, J. S., de Oliveira, M. M. & Panerai, R. B. (2012). Decompressive craniectomy: a meta-analysis of influences on intracranial pressure and cerebral perfusion pressure in the treatment of traumatic brain injury. *J Neurosurg*, *117*, 589-596.

[10] Bor-Seng-Shu, E., Figueiredo, E. G., Fonoff, E. T., Fujimoto, Y., Panerai, R. B. & Teixeira, M. J. (2013). Decompressive craniectomy and head injury: brain morphometry, ICP, cerebral hemodynamics, cerebral

microvascular reactivity, and neurochemistry. *Neurosurg Rev, 36*, 361-370.

[11] Brandt, L., Sonesson, B., Ljunggren, B. & Saveland, H. (1987). Ruptured middle cerebral artery aneurysm with intracerebral hemorrhage in younger patients appearing moribund: emergency operation? *Neurosurgery, 20*, 925-929.

[12] Buschemann, U., Yonekawa, Y., Fortunati, M., Cesnulis, E. & Keller, E. (2007). Decompressive hemicraniectomy in patients with subarachnoid hemorrhage and intractable intracranial hypertension. *Acta Neurochir (Wien), 149*, 59-65.

[13] Cho, D. Y., Chen, T. C. & Lee, H. C. (2003). Ultra-early decompressive craniectomy for malignant middle cerebral artery infarction. *Surg Neurol., 60*, 227-232.

[14] Claassen, J., Carhuapoma, J. R., Kreiter, K. T., Du, E. Y., Connolly, E. S. & Mayer, S. A. (2002). Global cerebral edema after subarachnoid hemorrhage: frequency, predictors, and impact on outcome. *Stroke, 33*, 1225–1232.

[15] D'Ambrosio, A. L., Sughrue, M. E., Yorgason, J. G., Mocco, J. D., Kreiter, K. T., Mayer, S. A., McKhann, G. M. & Connolly, E. S. (2005). Decompressive hemicraniectomy for poor-grade aneurysmal subarachnoid hemorrhage patients with associated intracerebral hemorrhage: clinical outcome and quality of life assessment. *Neurosurgery, 56*, 12-20.

[16] De Bonis, P., Pompucci, A., Mangiola, A., Rigante, L. & Anile, C. (2010). Post-traumatic hydrocephalus after decompressive craniectomy: an underestimated risk factor. *J Neurotrauma, 27*, 1965–1970.

[17] Dorfer, C., Frick, A., Knosp, E. & Gruber, A. (2010). Decompressive hemicraniectomy after aneurysmal subarachnoid hemorrhage. *World Neurosurg, 74*, 465–471.

[18] Guresir, E., Schuss, P., Vatter, H., Raabe, A., Seifert, V. & Beck, J. (2009). Decompressive craniectomy in subarachnoid hemorrhage. *Neurosurg Focus, 26(6)*, E4.

[19] Hauerberg, J., Eskesen, V. & Rosenorn, J. (1994). The prognostic significance of intracerebral hematoma as shown on CT scanning after aneurysmal subarachnoid hemorrhage. *Br J Neurosurg, 8*, 333-339.

[20] Hayashi, M., Kobayashi, H., Kawano, H., Yamamoto, S. & Maeda, T. (1984). Cerebral blood flow and ICP patterns in patients with communicating hydrocephalus after aneurysm rupture. *J Neurosurg, 61*, 30-36.

[21] Heuer, G., Smith, M., Elliott, J., Winn, H. & Leroux, P. (2004). Relationship between intracranial pressure and other clinical variables in patients with aneurysmal subarachnoid hemorrhage. *J Neurosurg*, *101*, 408-416.

[22] Jaeger, M., Soehle, M. & Meixensberger, J. (2003). Effects of decompressive craniotomy on brain tissue oxygen in patients with intracranial hypertension. *J Neurol Neurosurg Psychiatry*, *74*, 513-515.

[23] Janjua, N. & Mayer, S. A. (2003). Cerebral vasospasm after subarachnoid hemorrhage. *Curr Opin Crit Care*, *9*, 113–119.

[24] Jourdan, C., Convert, J., Mottolese, C., Bachour, E., Gharbi, S. & Artru, F. (1993). Evaluation of the clinical benefit of decompression hemicraniectomy in intracranial hypertension not controlled by medical treatment [in French]. *Neurochirurgie*, *39*, 304-310.

[25] Kakar, V., Nagaria, J. & John Kirkpatrick, P. (2009). The current status of decompressive craniectomy. *Br J Neurosurg*, *23*, 147–157.

[26] Kamiya, K., Inagawa, T., Yamamoto, M. & Monden, S. (1991). Subdural hematoma due to ruptured intracranial aneurysm. *Neurol Med Chir* (Tokyo), *31*, 82-86.

[27] Kaye, A. H. & Brownbill, D. (1981). Postoperative intracranial pressure in patients operated on for cerebral aneurysms following subarachnoid hemorrhage. *J Neurosurg*, *54*, 726-732.

[28] Kilincer, C., Asil, T., Utku, U., Hamamcioglu, M. K., Turgut, N., Hicdonmez, T., Simsek, O., Ekuklu, G. & Cobanoglu, S. (2005). Factors affecting the outcome of decompressive craniectomy for large hemispheric infarctions: A prospective cohort study. *Acta Neurochir* (Wien), *147*, 587–594.

[29] Koerbel, A., Ernemann, U. & Freudenstein, D. (2005). Acute subdural haematoma without subarachnoid hemorrhage caused by rupture of an internal carotid artery bifurcation aneurysm: case report and review of literature. *Br J Radiol*, *78*, 646-650.

[30] Kondziolka, D. & Fazl, M. (1988). Functional recovery after decompressive craniectomy for cerebral infarction. *Neurosurgery*, *23*, 143-147.

[31] Lagares, A., Putman, C. M. & Ogilvy, C. S. (2001). Posterior fossa decompression and clot evacuation for fourth ventricle hemorrhage after aneurysmal rupture: Case report. *Neurosurgery*, *49*, 208–211.

[32] Lazaridis, C. & Czosnyka, M. (2012). Cerebral blood flow, brain tissue oxygen, and metabolic effects of decompressive craniectomy. *Neurocrit Care*, *16*, 478-484.

[33] Lee, K. H., Lukovits, T. & Friedman, J. A. (2006). "Triple-H" therapy for cerebral vasospasm following subarachnoid hemorrhage. *Neurocrit Care*, *4*, 68–76.

[34] Le Roux, P. D., Elliott, J. P., Downey, L., Newell, D. W., Grady, M. S., Mayberg, M. R., Eskridge, J. M. & Winn, H. R. (1995). Improved outcome after rupture of anterior circulation aneurysms: a retrospective 10-year review of 224 good-grade patients. *J Neurosurg*, *83*, 394-402.

[35] Le Roux, P. D., Elliott, J. P., Newell, D. W., Grady, M. S. & Winn, H. R. (1996). Predicting outcome in poor-grade patients with subarachnoid hemorrhage: a prospective review of 159 aggressively managed cases. *J Neurosurg*, *85*, 39-49.

[36] Mokri, B. (2010). Orthostatic headaches in the syndrome of the trephined: resolution following cranioplasty. *Headache*, *50*, 1206–1211.

[37] Mori, K., Aoki, A., Yamamoto, T., Horinaka, N. & Maeda, M. (2001). Aggressive decompressive surgery in patients with massive hemispheric embolic cerebral infarction associated with severe brain swelling. *Acta Neurochir* (Wien), *143*, 483-491.

[38] Murad, A., Ghostine, S. & Colohan, A. R. (2011). Role of controlled lumbar CSF drainage for ICP control in aneurysmal SAH. *Acta Neurochir Suppl*, *110*, 183–187.

[39] Nagel, A., Graetz, D., Schink, T., Frieler, K., Sakowitz, O., Vajkoczy, P. & Sarrafzadeh, A. (2009). Relevance of intracranial hypertension for cerebral metabolism in aneurysmal subarachnoid hemorrhage. Clinical article. *J Neurosurg*, *111*, 94–101.

[40] Ohkuma, H., Shimamura, N., Fujita, S. & Suzuki, S. (2003). Acute subdural hematoma caused by aneurysmal rupture: incidence and clinical features. *Cerebrovasc Dis*, *16*, 171-173.

[41] Otani, N., Takasato, Y., Masaoka, H., Hayakawa, T., Yoshino, Y., Yatsushige, H., Miyawaki, H., Sumiyoshi, K., Chikashi, A., Takeuchi, S. & Suzuki, G. (2008). Surgical outcome following decompressive craniectomy for poor-grade aneurysmal subarachnoid hemorrhage in patients with associated massive intracerebral or Sylvian hematomas. *Cerebrovasc Dis*, *26*, 612-617.

[42] Otani, N., Takasato, Y., Masaoka, H., Hayakawa, T., Yoshino, Y., Yatsushige, H., Miyawaki, H., Sumiyoshi, K., Sugawara, T., Chikashi, A., Takeuchi, S. & Suzuki, G. (2011). Clinical characteristics and surgical outcomes of patients with aneurysmal subarachnoid hemorrhage and acute subdural hematoma undergoing decompressive craniectomy. *World Neurosurg*, *75*, 73-77.

[43] Polin, R. S., Shaffrey, M. E., Bogaev, C. A., Tisdale, N., Germanson, T., Bocchicchio, B. & Jane, J. A. (1997). Decompressive bifrontal craniectomy in the treatment of severe refractory posttraumatic cerebral edema. *Neurosurgery*, *41*, 84-94.

[44] Rahme, R., Weil, A. G., Sabbagh, M., Moumdjian, R., Bouthillier, A. & Bojanowski, M. W. (2010). Decompressive craniectomy is not an independent risk factor for communicating hydrocephalus in patients with increased intracranial pressure. *Neurosurgery*, *67*, 675–678.

[45] Rangel-Castillo, L. & Robertson, C. S. (2006). Management of intracranial hypertension. *Crit Care Clin*, *22*, 713–732.

[46] Reithmeier, T., Lohr, M., Rakos, P., Ketter, G. & Ernestus, R. L. (2005). Relevance of ICP and ptiO_2 for indication and timing of decompressive craniectomy in patients with malignant brain edema. *Acta Neurochir* (Wien), *147*, 947-952.

[47] Rosen, D. S. & Macdonald, R. L. (2005). Subarachnoid hemorrhage grading scales: a systematic review. *Neurocrit Care*, *2*, 110-118.

[48] Rosengart, A. J., Schultheiss, K. E., Tolentino, J. & Macdonald, R. L. (2007). Prognostic factors for outcome in patients with aneurysmal subarachnoid hemorrhage. *Stroke*, *38*, 2315–2321.

[49] Ryttlefors, M., Howells, T., Nilsson, P., Ronne-Engstrom, E. & Enblad, P. (2007). Secondary insults in subarachnoid hemorrhage: occurrence and impact on outcome and clinical deterioration. *Neurosurgery*, *61*, 704–714.

[50] Sandalcioglu, I. E., Schoch, B., Regel, J. P., Wanke, I., Gasser, T., Forsting, M., Stolke, D. & Wiedemayer, H. (2004). Does intraoperative aneurysm rupture influence outcome? Analysis of 169 patients. *Clin Neurol Neurosurg*, *106*, 88-92.

[51] Schirmer, C. M., Hoit, D. A. & Malek, A. M. (2007). Decompressive hemicraniectomy for the treatment of intractable intracranial hypertension after aneurysmal subarachnoid hemorrhage. *Stroke*, *38*, 987-992.

[52] Schmidt, J. M., Rincon, F., Fernandez, A., Resor, C., Kowalski, R. G., Claassen, J., Connolly, E. S., Fitzsimmons, B. F. & Mayer, S. A. (2007). Cerebral infarction associated with acute subarachnoid hemorrhage. *Neurocrit Care*, *7*, 10–17.

[53] Schwab, S., Steiner, T., Aschoff, A., Schwarz, S., Steiner, H. H., Jansen, O. & Hacke, W. (1998). Early hemicraniectomy in patients with complete middle cerebral artery infarction. *Stroke*, *29*, 1888-1893.

[54] Scozzafava, J., Brindley, P. G., Mehta, V. & Findlay, J. M. (2007). Decompressive bifrontal craniectomy for malignant intracranial pressure following anterior communicating artery aneurysm rupture: Two case reports. *Neurocrit Care*, *6*, 49–53.

[55] Seifert, V., Trost, H. A. & Stolke, D. (1990). Management morbidity and mortality in grade IV and V patients with aneurysmal subarachnoid hemorrhage. *Acta Neurochir* (Wien), *103*, 5-10.

[56] Shimoda, M., Oda, S., Mamata, Y., Tsugane, R. & Sato, O. (1997). Surgical indications in patients with an intracerebral hemorrhage due to ruptured middle cerebral artery aneurysm. *J Neurosurg*, *87*, 170-175.

[57] Smith, E. R., Carter, B. S. & Ogilvy, C. S. (2002). Proposed use of prophylactic decompressive craniectomy in poor-grade aneurysmal subarachnoid hemorrhage patients presenting with associated large sylvian hematomas. *Neurosurgery*, *51*, 117-124.

[58] Soehle, M., Chatfield, D. A., Czosnyka, M. & Kirkpatrick, P. J. (2007). Predictive value of initial clinical status, intracranial pressure and transcranial Doppler pulsatility after subarachnoid hemorrhage. *Acta Neurochir* (Wien), *149*, 575–583.

[59] Stiefel, M. F., Heuer, G. G., Smith, M. J., Bloom, S., Maloney-Wilensky, E., Gracias, V. H., Grady, M. S. & LeRoux, P. D. (2004). Cerebral oxygenation following decompressive hemicraniectomy for the treatment of refractory intracranial hypertension. *J Neurosurg*, *101*, 241-247.

[60] Stiver, S. I., Wintermark, M. & Manley, G. T. (2008). Reversible monoparesis following decompressive hemicraniectomy for traumatic brain injury. *J Neurosurg*, *109*, 245–254.

[61] Stiver, S. I. (2009). Complications of decompressive craniectomy for traumatic brain injury. *Neurosurg Focus*, *26*(6), E7.

[62] Stocchetti, N., Zanaboni, C., Colombo, A., Citerio, G., Beretta, L., Ghisoni, L., Zanier, E. R. & Canavesi, K. (2008). Refractory intracranial hypertension and "second-tier" therapies in traumatic brain injury. *Intensive Care Med*, *34*, 461–467.

[63] Takeuchi, S., Koike, T., Sasaki, O., Kamada, K., Tanaka, R. & Arai, H. (1989). Intracranial extradural pressure monitoring after direct operation on ruptured cerebral aneurysms. *Neurosurgery*, *24*, 878-883.

[64] Takeuchi, S., Nawashiro, H., Wada, K., Takasato, Y., Masaoka, H., Hayakawa, T., Nagatani, K., Otani, N., Osada, H. & Shima, K. (2013). Ventriculomegaly after decompressive craniectomy with hematoma

evacuation for large hemispheric hypertensive intracerebral hemorrhage. *Clin Neurol Neurosurg*, *115*, 317-322.

[65] Tokuda, Y., Inagawa, T., Katoh, Y., Kumano, K., Ohbayashi, N. & Yoshioka, H. (1995). Intracerebral hematoma in patients with ruptured cerebral aneurysms. *Surg Neurol*, *43*, 272-277.

[66] Tuzgen, S., Kucukyuruk, B., Aydin, S., Ozlen, F., Kizilkilic, O. & Abuzayed, B. (2012). Decompressive craniectomy in patients with cerebral infarction due to malignant vasospasm after aneurysmal subarachnoid hemorrhage. *J Neurosci Rural Pract*, *3*, 251–255.

[67] Ucar, T., Akyuz, M., Kazan, S. & Tuncer, R. (2005). Role of decompressive surgery in the management of severe head injuries: Prognostic factors and patient selection. *J Neurotrauma*, *22*, 1311–1318.

[68] van Gijn, J., Kerr, R. S. & Rinkel, G. J. E. (2007). Subarachnoid hemorrhage. *Lancet*, *369*(9558), 306–318.

[69] Wartenberg, K. E. (2011). Critical care of poor-grade subarachnoid hemorrhage. *Curr Opin Crit Care*, *17*, 85–93.

[70] Waziri, A., Fusco, D., Mayer, S. A., McKhann, G. M. 2nd & Connolly, E. S. Jr (2007). Postoperative hydrocephalus in patients undergoing decompressive hemicraniectomy for ischemic or hemorrhagic stroke. *Neurosurgery*, *61*, 489–493.

[71] Weir, B., Myles, T., Kahn, M., Maroun, F., Malloy, D., Benoit, B., McDermott, M., Cochrane, D., Mohr, G., Ferguson, G., et al (1984). Management of acute subdural hematomas from aneurysmal rupture. *Can J Neurol Sci*, *11*, 371-376.

[72] Yoshimoto, Y., Wakai, S., Satoh, A. & Hirose, Y. (1999). Intraparenchymal and intrasylvian haematomas secondary to ruptured middle cerebral artery aneurysms: prognostic factors and therapeutic considerations. *Br J Neurosurg*, *13*, 18-24.

In: Subarachnoid Hemorrhage
Editor: Linda R. Gray

ISBN: 978-1-63463-492-2

Chapter 8

Subarachnoid Hemorrhage: Postoperative Management

Eiji Isotani, MD, PhD*

Department of Emergency and Critical Care Medicine, Tokyo Women's Medical University Medical Center, Tokyo, Japan

Abstract

Introduction: Volume management is crucial in intensive care, however, in some patients it is very hard to achieve optimal water balance. Subarachnoid hemorrhage (SAH) patient is a representative example. Cardiopulmonary complications are common after SAH: neurogenic pulmonary edema, cardiac failure, and so on.

Triple H therapy is a standard management after SAH, but it also has adverse effects; pulmonary edema, increased intracranial pressure, hyponatremia, sepsis and so on. We have just finished the multicenter prospective cohort study about cardiopulmonary function after SAH. We describe herein the novel goal directed therapy after SAH.

Material and Methods: This multicenter prospective cohort study analyzed the cardiopulmonary functions of 204 patients after SAH by PiCCO plus™ monitoring over a period of two weeks.

* Eiji Isotani, MD, PhD: Department of Emergency and Critical Care Medicine, Tokyo Women's Medical University Medical Center East 2-1-10 Nishi-Ogu, Arakawa-ku, Tokyo 113-8567, Japan. Tel: +81-3-3810-1111. E-mail: isotaner@dnh.twmu.ac.jp.

Results: Triple H therapy did not decrease the occurrence of delayed cerebral ischemia (DCI).

The risk factors of DCI on PiCCO plus™ monitoring were low cardiac index (CI), high systemic vascular resistance (SVRI), and low global end-diastolic volume index (GEDI). The cut-off value of GEDI was 822mL/m^2 to decrease the occurrence of DCI and 921 mL/m^2 to increase the occurrence of pulmonary edema.

Conclusions: Triple H therapy did not decrease the occurrence of DCI after SAH. We suggested the novel goal directed therapy to prevent DCI by PiCCO plus™ monitoring. This novel goal directed therapy is to keep the GEDI between 822mL/m^2 and 921 mL/m^2.

Keywords: Goal directed therapy, delayed cerebral ischemia, global end-diastolic volume index

Introduction

Volume management is crucial in intensive care, however, in some patients it is very hard to achieve optimal water balance. Subarachnoid hemorrhage (SAH) patient is a representative example. Cardiopulmonary complications are common after SAH: neurogenic pulmonary edema, cardiac failure, and so on [1].

Triple H therapy (hypertension, hypervolemia, hemodilution) is a standard management after SAH [2], but it also has adverse effects; pulmonary edema, increased intracranial pressure, hyponatremia, sepsis and so on [3].

Therefore, we have to assess triple H therapy, and, if it does not work for preventing delayed cerebral ischemia (DCI), we must establish the new volume management strategy to reduce DCI onset.

Medical students learn Frank-Starling's law in the physiology class of medical school. This law explains that the cardiac muscle is pulled longer, stronger the tension is produced. Figure 1 shows the Frank-Starling's law of the heart. GEDI is global end-diastolic volume index of 4 chambers of the heart. High GEDI means hypervolemia, low GEDI means hypovolemia or dehydration. Increased GEDI results in the increase of cardiac index (CI), however, this positive correlation is not linear.

After achieving the adequate preload, the excess infusion causes only minimal increase of CI resulting in the congestion of pulmonary circulation. This congestion results in the increase of extravascular lung water index (ELWI). In short, CI and ELWI are important parameters to determine the appropriate preload. In case of cardiac failure, this Frank-Starling's curve shifts downward and the appropriate preload shifts to left.

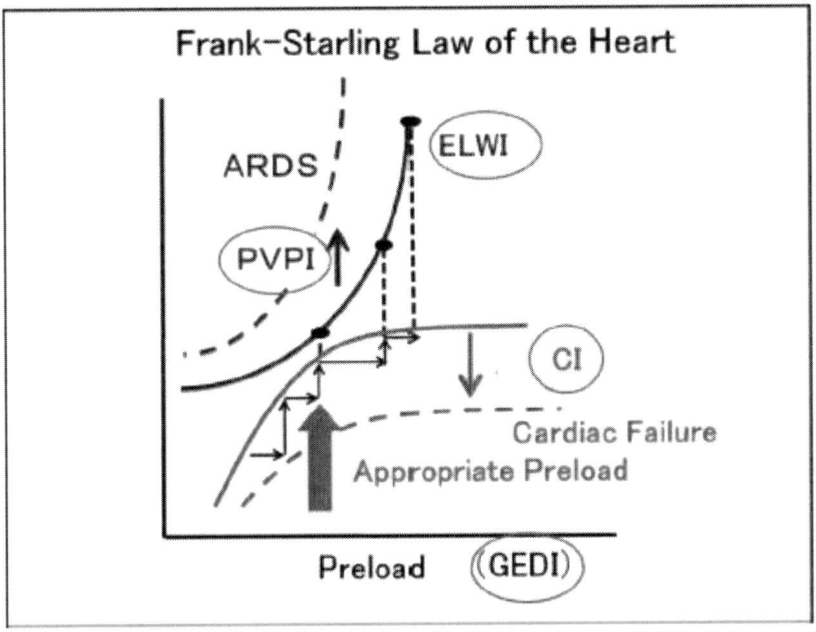

GEDI: Global End-diastolic Volume Index, CI: Cardiac Index, ELWI; Extravascular Lung Water Index, PVPI: Pulmonary Vascular Permeability Index.

Figure 1. Frank-Starling law of the heart.

In case of ARDS with high pulmonary permeability index (PVPI), the appropriate preload also shifts to left. Then in case of cardiac failure or ARDS, we reduce the fluid infusion.

PiCCO plus™ (PULSION, Germany) monitoring can provide these important parameters: CI, GEDI, ELWI and PVPI. The measurement of these parameters is available by the installation of central venous line and intra-arterial PiCCO™ catheter with thermistor (Figure 2).

We have just finished the multicenter prospective cohort study about cardiopulmonary function after SAH by using PiCCO plus™ (SAH PiCCO study). We describe herein the novel goal directed therapy after SAH obtained by the products from SAH PiCCO study.

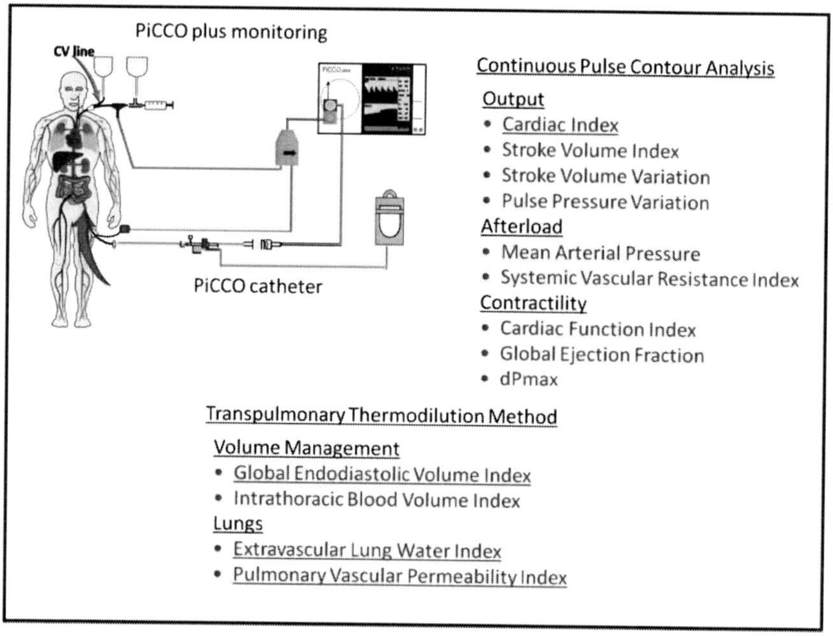

Figure 2. PiCCO plus™ monitoring.

Material and Methods

Two hundreds and four patients from 9 institutions were enrolled into this study. On admission, all patients were examined using computed tomography (CT), and their conditions were classified according the World Federation of Neurological Surgeons scale for severity [4] and Fisher group criteria for CT findings [5]. Patients were included if they had a ruptured cerebral aneurysm documented by cerebral angiography or 3-dimensional angiography. The exclusion criteria were (1) less than 15 years of age, (2) disappearance of brain stem reflexes, (3) pregnancy, and (4) severe cardiopulmonary dysfunction requiring percutaneous cardio-pulmonary support.

After ruptured aneurysmal obliteration, each patient was managed under PiCCO plus monitoring over a period of two weeks. Briefly, each patient was installed the central venous line and the intra-arterial PiCCO™ catheter with the thermistor. Both catheters were connected to the PiCCO plus™ for continuous monitoring of cardiac output, contractility, and afterload.

Transpulmonary thermodilution was performed at least once a day to monitor volume management and lung water. Measurements were obtained by injecting 15mL of an ice-cold saline bolus into the superior vena cava, with subsequent detection by the thermistor of the intra-arterial PiCCO™ catheter. Thermodilution curves according to the Stewart-Hamilton principle were recorded from the PiCCO™ catheter to allow estimations of CI (normal range, 3.0~5.0 L/min per square meter), GEDI (680~800 mL/m^2) [6], ELWI (3.0~10.0 mL/kg) [7], PVPI (1.0~3.0), and SVRI (1700~2400 dyn·s/cm^5 per square meter). Pulmonary edema (PE) was defined as a PaO_2/FiO_2 ratio<300 and bilateral infiltrative shadows observed on chest radiography. Data were collected into SAH PiCCO databank.

Data were presented as either the mean ± SE or the median (interquartile range, IQR), as appropriate. The groups were compared using Student t test or the Mann-Whitney U test as appropriate. Categorical comparisons were made using the chi-square test. We used Spearman's correlation coefficient (r) to examine relationships between variables. A repeated measures analysis was used to compare the distributions of outcomes during the entire study period. To determine the threshold values, receiver operating characteristic (ROC) curves were generated and used the Youden index for GEDI to associate with DCI and severe PE. The area under the ROC (AUC) was evaluated and presented with a 95% CI. Kaplan-Meier plots with log rank statistics and a Cox proportional hazards model were used to assess the outcomes for developing DCI and PE. A p value of less than 0.05 was considered significant for all statistical tests. Statistical analyses were performed using SPSS 17.0 for Windows (IBM, Armonk, NY).

Results

I. Assessment of Triple H Therapy

One hundred and four patients (59%) received triple H therapy and 71 patients (35%) suffered from DCI. There were no significant differences in age, sex, or SAH severity between the triple-H and control (non-triple H) groups at admission. Although there was no difference in dobutamine or albumin use, there were higher rates of clipping and fasudil® infusion in the triple-H group than in the control group. In addition, a greater amount of fluid was administrated to the triple-H group than the control group during the study period as analyzed by the generalized linear mixed model (GLMM) (p <

0.001). Although the MAP was significantly higher in the triple-H group than in the control group (p = 0.005), no significant differences were observed in GEDI (p = 0.81), fluid balance (p = 0.15), CVP (p = 0.18), cardiac index (CI) (p = 0.62), hematocrit (p = 0.71), or extravascular lung water index (p = 0.70) as analyzed by the GLMM. Figure 3 [8] shows the Kaplan–Meier curve for the occurrence of DCI following SAH, and no significant difference was observed between the 2 groups (log-rank test: χ^2 = 0.96, p = 0.33). The results of the Cox proportional hazards model indicate that the prophylactic triple-H therapy was not significantly associated with the occurrence of DCI, even after adjustment for other confounding factors. In short, triple H therapy did not reduce the incidence of DCI.

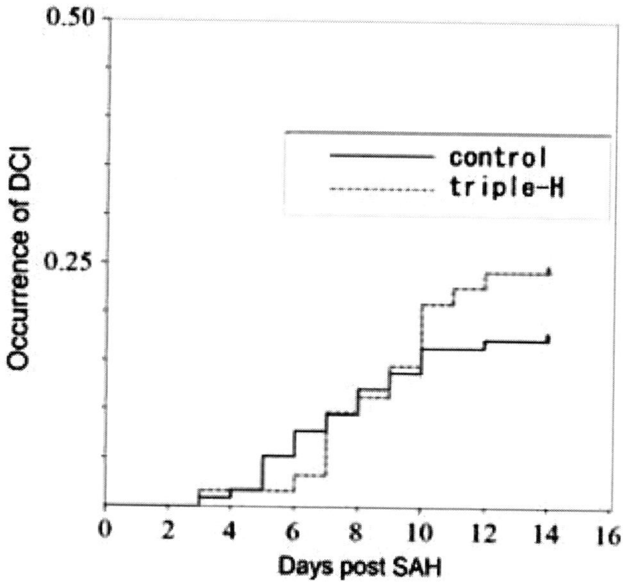

Cited from reference [8].

Figure 3. Triple H therapy did not reduce the incidence of DCI.

II. Independent Risk Factors for DCI

The mean onset day of DCI was day 8.0±3.3. GEDI from days 1 to 14 was slightly above the normal limit in the non-DCI group and was significantly lower in the DCI group on day 3 to 5 compared with the non-DCI group (p=0.0053, 0.048, and 0.048, respectively). ELWI and PVPI were within the normal range in both groups during the entire study period. CI was significantly lower in the DCI group on days 3, 4, and 6 (p=0.020, 0.042, and 0.0026, respectively). SVRI was significantly higher in the DCI group on days 3 to 7, and day 9 (p=0.049, 0.029, 0.036, 0.00031, 0.0093, and p=0.028, respectively).

In multivariate analysis, the independent risk factors of delayed cerebral ischemia on PiCCO plus monitoring were low CI (odds ratio, 0.602; 95%CI, 0.404-0.897; p=0.013), high SVRI (odds ratio, 1.001; 95% CI, 1.000-1.002; p=0.003), and low GEDI (odds ratio, 0.997; 95% CI, 0.995-1.000, p=0.023) on days 3 to 6 after SAH (Table 1) [9].

Table 1. Risk factors for delayed cerebral ischemia

Variables	OR	95%CI	p Value
Age	1.01	0.98-1.04	0.59
Gender (Female)	2.11	0.87-5.15	0.1
Pulmonary edema	1.02	0.41-2.50	0.97
Clipping	0.9	0.42-1.93	0.78
SAH severity	1.23	0.56-2.67	0.61
Cardiac index	0.6	0.40-0.90	0.013
Global end-diastolic volume index	0.997	0.995-1.000	0.023
Systemic vascular resistance index	1.001	1.000-1.002	0.003
Extravascular lung water index	0.93	0.83-1.04	0.2
Pulmonary vascular permeability index	0.898	0.43-1.89	0.78

III. Goal Directed Therapy after Subarachnoid Hemorrhage

GEDI on days 3 to 5 ROC curves used to associate with DCI indicated that the AUC was 0.66 (95%CI, 0.56-0.76). The GEDI threshold that best associated with DCI was 822 mL/m^2 (73% sensitivity, 64% specificity). Kaplan-Meier curve for the occurrence of DCI indicated that the low-GEDI group showed a significantly higher prevalence of DCI than the high-GEDI group (31.6% vs 9.4%; p<0.001). There were no significant differences between the two groups for CVP, CI, hematocrit, ELWI, or other variables during the study period.

We observed no significant differences in GEDI within either the PE patients group or the non-PE patient group during the entire study period. However, the GEDI was significantly higher in the PE group than the non-PE group in each phase. Using the Cox proportional hazards model, we found that GEDI on days 4 to 7 was significant variable that associated with PE occurrence (hazard ratio, the risk increase for every 100 in scale, 1.31; 95% CI, 1.02-1.71; p=0.03). Furthermore, a significant correlation was identified between GEDI and ELWI (r=0.46; p<0.001).

The GEDI ROC curves used to associate with the occurrence of PE indicated that the AUC was 0.77(95% CI, 0.69-0.85). The GEDI threshold that best associated with severe PE was 921 mL/m^2 (72% sensitivity, 71% specificity). The Kaplan-Meier curve for the occurrence of severe PE indicated that the prevalence of severe PE was significantly higher in the high-GEDI group than in the low-GEDI-group (43.6% vs 17.9%; p<0.001).

In short, the cut-off value of GEDI was 822mL/m^2 to increase the occurrence of DCI and 921 mL/m^2 to increase the occurrence of PE (Figure 4) [10].

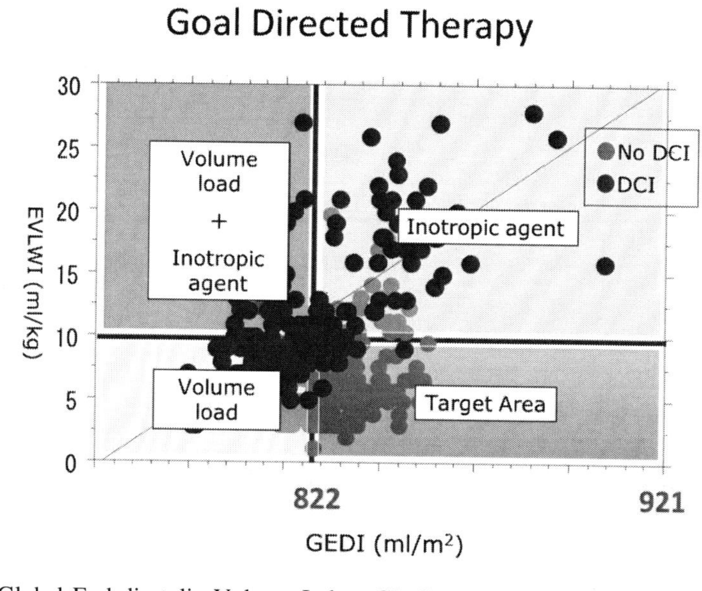

GEDI: Global End-diastolic Volume Index, CI: Cardiac Index, ELWI; Extravascular Lung Water Index.

Figure 4. Goal directed therapy after subarachnoid hemorrhage.

Discussion

The results of the current prospective multicenter study indicate that prophylactic administration of triple-H therapy, in the absence of treatment goals for the hemodynamic variables, was not associated with improved clinical outcomes.

Although a greater amount of fluid and a higher MAP were observed in the triple-H group, no significant difference was observed between the groups in CI or GEDI, a quantitative indicator of intravascular volume, despite the expectation that a significantly higher GEDI/CI would be observed in the treatment group than in the control group.

I. Assessment of Triple H Therapy

Although limited evidence from clinical trials supports the use of prophylactic triple-H therapy [11, 12, 13], it continues to be used in a number of institutions globally [14, 15, 16]. There have been few well-designed prospective studies with adequate sample sizes to provide strong evidence for the benefits of this therapeutic approach [17, 18]. The results of the current multicenter study were consistent with previous studies in that the use of prophylactic triple-H therapy following aneurysm surgery did not improve the clinical outcomes, including DCI [17, 18]. Previous studies based fluid therapy decisions on CVP, which is currently considered a poor indicator for intravascular volume status [19, 20]. In the present study, we assessed hypovolemia using more accurate methods, including the measurement of GEDI using the PiCCO plus™ system [8].

II. Independent Risk Factors for DCI

The characteristic hemodynamics of patients with SAH associated with DCI were equivalent to hypovolemia through a combination of hemodynamics specific to afterload mismatch cardiac failure before the onset of DCI with a significantly lower CI, a significantly higher SVRI, and a significantly lower GEDI [9]. The current study indicates the association between GEDI and DCI. We reported an association between low GEDI and the onset of DCI and identified a quantitative discrimination GEDI threshold (<822 mL/m^2) for predicting DCI [10]; this value was slightly higher than the published GEDI reference range (680–800 mL/m^2) [20], suggesting that the results are consistent with the concept of a hypervolemic goal for triple-H therapy. We, therefore, hypothesized in the present study that triple-H prophylaxis would increase the GEDI (i.e., >822 mL/m^2) and may prevent the onset of DCI following an SAH. However, triple-H prophylaxis in the absence of a strict protocol or goal-directed therapy may not increase the GEDI; therefore, we did not detect differences in the clinical outcome between the groups. The use of individually optimized GEDI-directed therapy might have changed the outcome [10]. The present study facilitates the need for additional GEDI-directed interventional studies (i.e., methods to increase GEDI) and provides the basis for future work to improve the management algorithms for SAH patients with the aim of preventing DCI.

III. Goal Directed Therapy after Subarachnoid Hemorrhage

Management of hemodynamic status with the goal of preventing not only hypovolemia but also hypervolemia is clinically important. Fluid management is an extremely important component of treatment for patients with SAH because of the high risk of potential fluid imbalance–related complications, including DCI and neurogenic PE. The current study also indicates a correlation between GEDI and severe PE. The findings of the present study suggest that GEDI is correlated with both the onset of DCI (threshold < 822 mL/m^2) and severe PE (threshold > 921 mL/m^2) [10].

A quantitative discrimination threshold associated with severe PE was GEDI greater than 921 mL/m^2, considering that inappropriate intravascular fluid accumulation may result in the accumulation of extravascular lung water, which manifests clinically as PE. Thus, ELWI and GEDI can be used as indicators for “when to stop” fluid administration.

Conclusion

Triple H therapy did not decrease the occurrence of DCI after SAH. We suggested the novel goal directed therapy to prevent DCI by PiCCO plus monitoring. This novel goal directed therapy is to keep the GEDI between 822mL/m^2 and 921 mL/m^2.

References

[1] Wood, J. H., Fleischer, A. S. Observations during hypervolemic hemodilution of patients with acute focal cerebral ischemia. *JAMA* 248: 2999-304, 1982.

[2] Kosnik, E. J., Hunt, W. E. Postoperative hypertension in the management of patients with intracranial arterial aneurysms. *J. Neurosurg.* 45: 148-154, 1976.

[3] Friedman, J. A., Pichelmann, M. A., Piepgras, D. G., et al. Pulmonary complications of aneurismal subarachnoid hemorrhage. *Neurosurgery*. 2003;52:1025-1031.

[4] Drake, C. G., Hunt, W. E., Sano, K. Report of World Federation of Neurological Surgeons Committee on a universal subarachnoid hemorrhage grading scale. *J. Neurosurg*. 1988;68:985-986.

[5] Fisher, C. M., Kistler, J. P., Davis, J. M. Relation of cerebral vasospasm to subarachnoid hemorrhage visualized by computerized tomographic scanning. *Neurosurgery*. 1980;6:1-9.

[6] Sakka, S. G., Rühl, C. C., Pfeiffer, U. J., et al. Assessment of cardiac preload and extravascular lung water by single transpulmonary thermodilution. *Intensive Care Med*. 2000;26:180-187.

[7] Newman, E. V., Merrell, M., Genecin, A., et al. The dye dilution method for describing the central circulation. An analysis of factors shaping the time-concentration curves. *Circulation*. 1951;4:735-746.

[8] Tagami, T., Kuwamoto, K., Watanabe, A., et al. Effect of Triple-H Prophylaxis on Global End-Diastolic Volume and Clinical Outcomes in Patients with Aneurysmal Subarachnoid Hemorrhage. *Neurocrit. Care*. 2014 May 28. [Epub. ahead of print].

[9] Yoneda, H., Nakamura, T., Shirao, S., et al. Multicenter Prospective Cohort Study on Volume Management After Subarachnoid Hemorrhage: Hemodynamic Changes According to Severity of Subarachnoid Hemorrhage and Cerebral Vasospasm. *Stroke*. 44(8):2155-61, 2013.

[10] Tagami, T., Kuwamoto, K., Watanabe, A., et al. Optimal Range of Global End-Diastolic Volume for Fluid Management After Aneurysmal Subarachnoid Hemorrhage: A Multicenter Prospective Cohort Study. *Critical Care Medicine*, Volume 42(6), p. 1348-1356, 2014.

[11] Rinkel, G. J., Feigin, V. L., Algra, A., van Gijn, J. Circulatory volume expansion therapy for aneurysmal subarachnoid hemorrhage. *Cochrane Database Syst. Rev.* 2004:CD000483.

[12] Diringer, M. N., Bleck, T. P., Claude Hemphill, J. III, et al. Critical care management of patients following aneurysmal subarachnoid hemorrhage: recommendations from the Neurocritical Care Society's Multidisciplinary Consensus Conference. *Neurocrit. Care.* 2011;15:211-40.

[13] Treggiari, M. M., Walder, B., Suter, P. M., Romand, J. A. Systematic review of the prevention of delayed ischemic neurological deficits with hypertension, hypervolemia, and hemodilution therapy following subarachnoid hemorrhage. *J. Neurosurg.* 2003;98:978-84.

[14] Sakowitz, O. W., Raabe, A., Vucak, D., Kiening, K. L., Unterberg, A. W. Contemporary management of aneurysmal subarachnoid hemorrhage in Germany: results of a survey among 100 neurosurgical departments. *Neurosurgery.* 2006;58:137-45.

[15] Stevens, R. D., Naval, N. S., Mirski, M. A., Citerio, G., Andrews, P. J. Intensive care of aneurysmal subarachnoid hemorrhage: an international survey. *Intensive Care Med.* 2009;35:1556-66.

[16] Meyer, R., Deem, S., Yanez, N. D., Souter, M., Lam, A., Treggiari, M. M. Current practices of triple-H prophylaxis and therapy in patients with subarachnoid hemorrhage. *Neurocrit. Care.* 2011;14:24-36.

[17] Egge, A., Waterloo, K., Sjoholm, H., Solberg, T., Ingebrigtsen, T., Romner, B. Prophylactic hyperdynamic postoperative fluid therapy after aneurysmal subarachnoid hemorrhage: a clinical, prospective, randomized, controlled study. *Neurosurgery.* 2001;49:593-605 discussion 605-596.

[18] Lennihan, L., Mayer, S. A., Fink, M. E., et al. Effect of hypervolemic therapy on cerebral blood flow after subarachnoid hemorrhage: a randomized controlled trial. *Stroke.* 2000;31:383-91.

[19] Marik, P. E., Cavallazzi, R. Does the central venous pressure predict fluid responsiveness? An updated meta-analysis and a plea for some common sense. *Crit. Care Med.* 2013;41:1774-81.

[20] Lazaridis, C. Advanced hemodynamic monitoring: principles and practice in neurocritical care. *Neurocrit. Care.* 2012;16:163-9.

[21] Goepfert, M. S., Richter, H. P., Eulenburg, C. Z., et al. Individually optimized hemodynamic therapy reduces complications and length of stay in the intensive care unit: a prospective, randomized controlled trial. *Anesthesiology.* 2013;119:824-36.

Index

D

E

F

G

H

L

M

Q

R

S

T

U

V

W

X